MIND & MEMBRAIN

HEAD INJURIES AND MENTAL HEALTH – A NEW APPROACH TO DIAGNOSIS AND TREATMENT

JOANNA WILDY

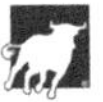

Matador
Unit E2 Airfield Business Park,
Harrison Road, Market Harborough,
Leicestershire. LE16 7UL
Tel: 0116 2792299
Email: books@troubador.co.uk
Web: www.troubador.co.uk/matador
Twitter: @matadorbooks

ISBN 978 1 80313 515 1

British Library Cataloguing in Publication Data.
A catalogue record for this book is available from the British Library.

Printed and bound in the UK by TJ Books LTD, Padstow, Cornwall
Typeset in 11pt Caslon Pro by Troubador Publishing Ltd, Leicester, UK

Matador is an imprint of Troubador Publishing Ltd

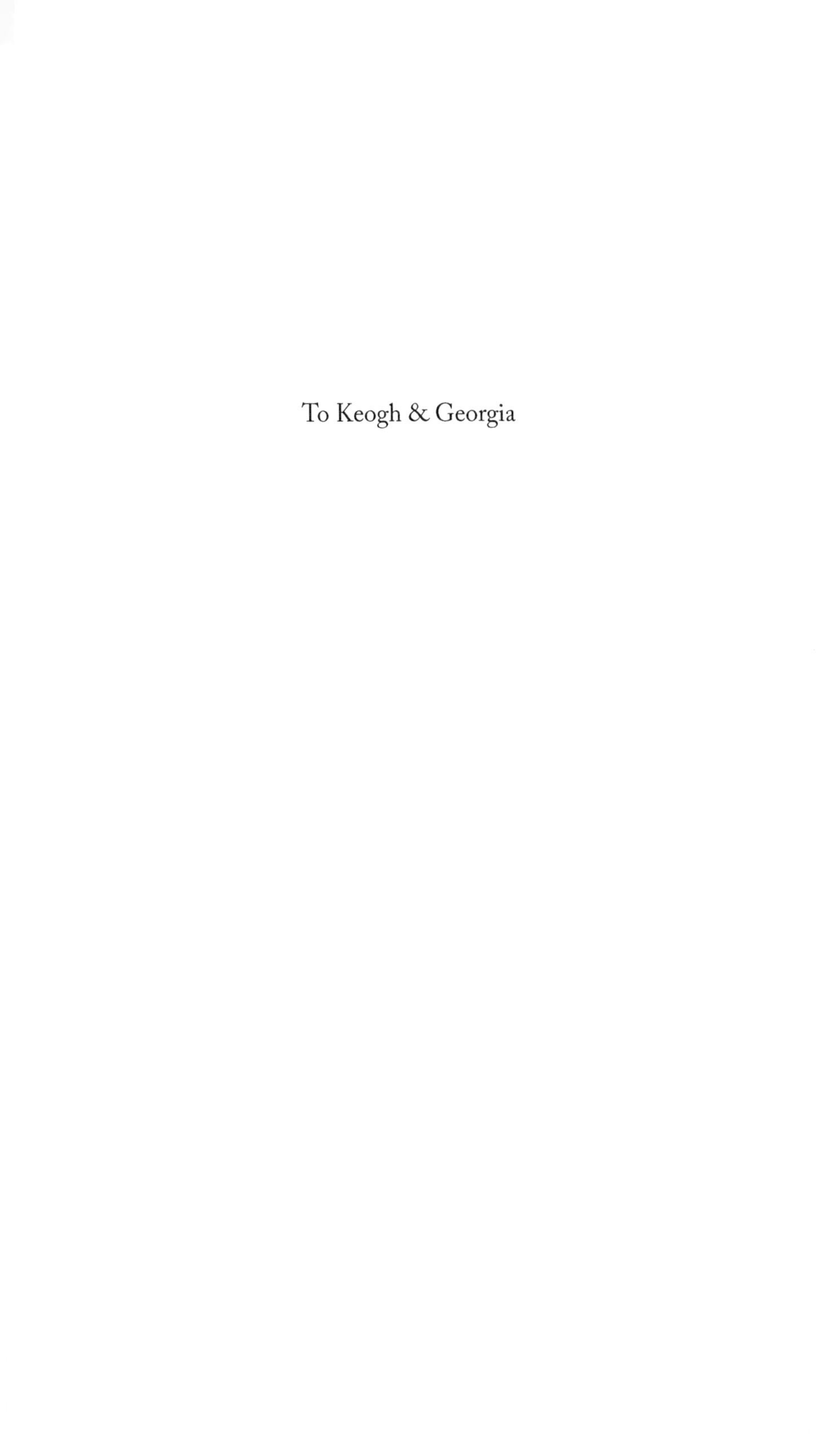

To Keogh & Georgia

CONTENTS

AUTHOR'S FOREWORD

The title of this book '*Mind & Membrain*' describes the direct relationship between the mind, the health of the brain and the state of the membrane system that lines the skull and envelops the brain. The technical name for this overlooked membrane is the *dura mater*, or dura for short. The dura is a living, reactive and responsive system that has a strong influence on the behaviour and long-term health of its occupant, the brain. Any impact to the head, however slight, can cause a disturbance of the dura and in turn of the brain. Mental health problems can be a consequence – and these problems can be successfully treated. As such, the brain-membrane link deserves some long overdue attention!

The person whose pioneering work laid the foundation for this concept was William Garner Sutherland (1873–1954). WGS, as he is known, was one of the second ever generation of osteopaths to emerge from the USA in the early 20th century. He stood apart from the rest of his colleagues whose interests followed those of the 'founding father' of osteopathy, Andrew Taylor Still (1828–1917), namely the study of the spine and general body.[1] WGS, by contrast, was fixated on the skull. It was a lifetime's work for him – tireless, relentless anatomical exploration and self-study over decades.

Doubting the accepted view that the skull is a single, fixed and solid structure, Sutherland painstakingly prised apart the 22 individual bones of which it is composed. He did this with tweezers, not a crowbar as one might suppose, revealing the extraordinary intricacies and delicate engineering of the different joint lines sitting between the collective bones of the skull. Situated directly beneath this remarkable piece of engineering and connected with it via anchorage points lies a dynamic cranial membrane: the dura mater. The dura is an active, responsive system. It is the state of this membrane system, in response to the positional relationships of the different cranial bones, that influences the health of the brain for reasons that will become clearly apparent.

On voicing his discoveries to fellow students and colleagues, WGS was ridiculed. Undeterred, he persevered with his research, pushing his independent studies on relentlessly. "I undertook" he writes, "to devise experiments, duplicating the effects of traumatic events as precisely as I could...." His scientific equipment over the years included an American football helmet, a wooden butter bowl and baseball catching mitts, plus an assortment of chamois leathers, bandages and flexible rulers. He adapted his equipment for each experiment and took to wearing his self-constructed skull-exploring equipment for days at a time. He used the various items to exert pressure from outside-in onto different parts of his skull, thus mimicking the results of various types of head injury. He did this to self-observe how a continuous pressure on the different areas of the cranium influenced his physical health – and also his mental health.[2]

The effects he experienced were extraordinary, not only physiologically, but also psychologically: "One experiment" he records, "left me ready for a stay in a mental hospital...."

In 1988, nearly a century after WGS began his experiments on the skull, I completed four years of undergraduate study to become an osteopath in the UK and decided to enrol on the postgraduate programme for osteopathy in the cranial field; that is, osteopathy which has a particular interest in the head. This is the specialist field that has developed over the last century directly from WGS's work.

And so begins my own story – a continuation of a particular aspect of William Garner Sutherland's work: his discoveries relating the skull and underlying membrane system – which together constitute the housing, the environment, of the brain – to mental health.

My postgraduate course started with a five-day programme of anatomy lectures, with practical hands-on sessions among the students after each lesson. Anyone who works in this field will appreciate that this is a lot of time to have untrained hands probing your head and face. The intensity of the course took its toll and by the end of the five-day introductory course I was starting to feel mentally very unwell.

From the start of secondary school, I had struggled with what I call low-grade depression and fluctuating moods. I found life from eleven to eighteen purgatory, if I am honest, but had always put it down to various understandable factors in my life – the see-saw of intense emotions and experiences typical of the teenage years.

During my twenties I suffered again from exaggerated mood swings; these were emerging as my nemesis. However, after that five-day introduction to the postgraduate programme, the depression and the struggle with my feelings that I had experienced on and off became significantly worse. The episodes were intensive and dark and went on for months. Eventually I decided to withdraw from the course.

A few months later, by sheer good fortune, I found someone who could help me. I was working as a tutor and practitioner at the British School of Osteopathy when I came across Carol Plumridge, a colleague with a great deal of experience in cranial osteopathy. She offered me a treatment. It took just one session with her skilled hands working on my head for the persistent depression that I had been experiencing since the fateful course to lift. The darkness turned to light, the world changed from a hostile to a friendly place and the treacle that I had been walking through turned to air. The whole experience made me understand the strength of this hands-on cranial therapeutic intervention: a power for bad when one is treated incorrectly, but a power for the utmost good if treated well.

Three years on from my initial attempt, I enrolled again on the postgraduate programme for osteopathy in the cranial field. I was by now far more observant and aware of my vulnerability and I found I could become the objective observer as untrained hands practised their poorly managed skills on my head. Strangely enough, a bad reaction to a hands-on experience can reveal more than a positive reaction. When you feel better from a treatment, there is a tendency to forget the initial discomfort. If you feel worse after a treatment, you remember it. And there it was, day four, with twelve sets of untrained hands exploring one after the other the anatomy of my viscero-cranium, better known as my face.

I left early that day, aware of a mighty setback in terms of my emotional health. The darkness, hostility and sense of wading through treacle had descended on me yet again, like the sudden onset of a tropical storm. A switch from bright sunshine to murky deluge in the shortest space of time.

This time I knew exactly what to do. I located Carol, travelled across London to her practice and had an osteopathic treatment. I put what felt like my battered self in her safe hands and – immediately – spirits restored; depression lifted.

I have a history of trauma to my face. To this day it sits there, visibly. I have (though not everyone notices it) a bumpy nose and chipped front teeth, a result of three major traumas to my face at the ages of two, six and eight. When I was two I fell down the stairs, from the very top to bottom, and my nose took the brunt. I have no memory of this event. I remember the second one; I was sitting in the saddle at the very front of the playground rocking horse when a group of older children jumped on the back and turned it into a bucking bronco! My brand new front teeth slammed down on the head of the horse. Not much pain until I showed my Mum who told me that it would be OK but I would never be beautiful – then I cried. The final trauma was running fast and falling hard, face first onto a London pavement.

When I was eleven, these traumas culminated in a hideous operation on my nose and the nasal fossa (the cavity that air flows through) that sits behind it. As the years passed, beyond the obvious cosmetic consequences to my nose and teeth, I was not aware of any lasting physical legacy from either the original injuries or the painful surgical procedures meant to fix them. And it certainly never occurred to me that they might affect my mental state – my thoughts, moods and feelings.

I think back to my gloomy late childhood and teenage years. They stand in very sharp contrast to my cheerful early childhood up to age eleven. What separates these two parts of my timeline was my face and the area behind it being attacked by a drill. No one would ever consider such an event, amongst all the other events in one's life, as a contributory factor to a mental health problem – I didn't myself at the time. But, in retrospect, when I considered the effect on my own mental health of students' untrained hands on my face, and the instant response to a skilled correction by a cranial osteopath, I realised that the historical damage to my face and skull had left its physical legacy which had a substantial influence on the stability of my mental health.

Once I understood how the skull and mental health were linked, I began to pay as much attention to my patients' emotional health as I did to their physical aches and pains. Osteopaths who like me are trained in the cranial field are a subsection of the worldwide osteopathic profession. I am one of about five thousand osteopaths currently registered in the UK. Despite the name, a cranial osteopath, like any osteopath, treats the whole body *and* the head. Osteopathy in its intended format is not about treating the musculoskeletal system. It is about using the musculoskeletal system as a tool to have a far-reaching impact on the health of the whole body. During my more than thirty years of practice I have become ever more convinced from the treatment outcomes that in certain patients with mental health problems it is the physical housing of the brain – the skull and importantly the underlying membrane system, the dura – that is the problem.

I have been fortunate to work in this field and thus to have discovered the extraordinary benefit of a specific hands-on treatment approach when I was experiencing mental distress. There are so many others like me who have suffered head injury or face trauma and subsequent mental health issues who do not know where to look for help. The physical origin of their condition involving the dural membrane is simply not recognised in the medical world. Despite all the kind attention of GPs, psychotherapists and psychiatrists and a host of other treatments, including all the self-help on offer, nothing has really worked for them. Medication has no lasting impact on their mental state, and on top of that disappointment they have to tolerate the side-effects of the drugs (weight gain, "walking around in a fog", a metallic taste in the mouth, disturbed sleep…) and then, finally, the withdrawal effects are often even worse.

It is not an uncommon story.

This book offers a story with a different ending.

Jo Wildy
Kew, 2022

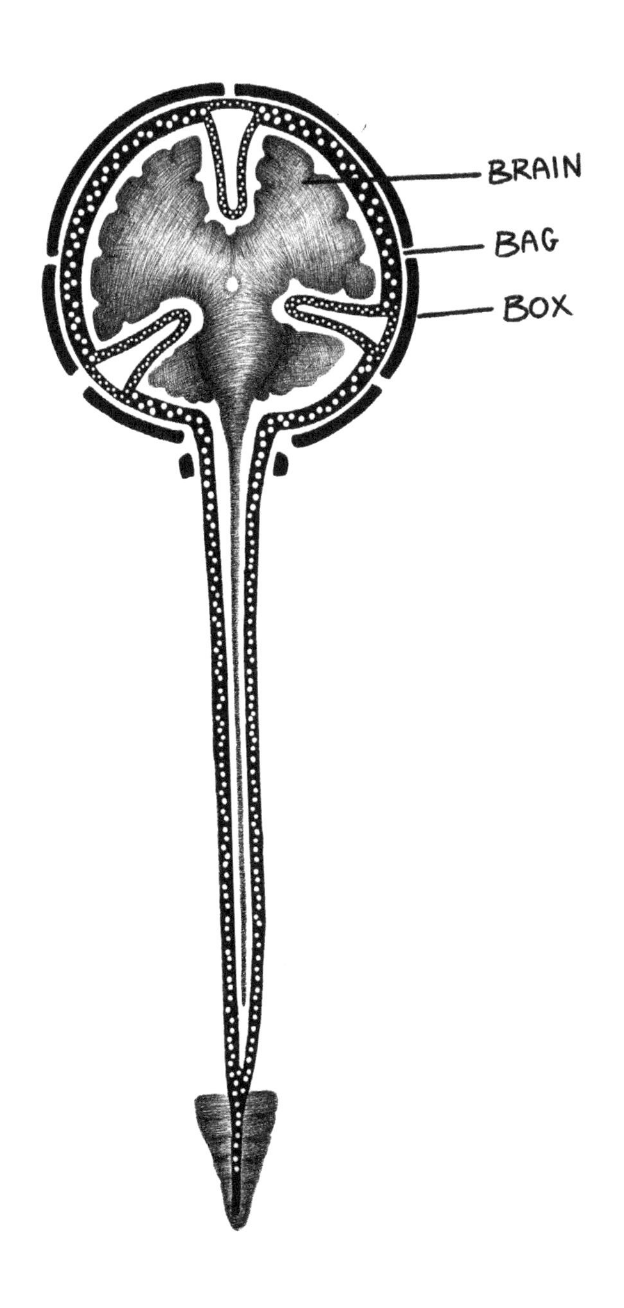
BRAIN
BAG
BOX

INTRODUCTION

Amy

Amy* was thirteen when her parents brought her for a consultation. There was a dramatic and ongoing deterioration in Amy's behaviour. Several months earlier she had started acting aggressively and at times violently towards various friends, out of character and for absolutely no reason – and the problem was escalating. Amy's parents were at the point of taking the psychiatrist's advice to medicate her.

In thirty years of practice I have examined and treated thousands of patients, many with mental health problems. I examined Amy by holding and sensing the different parts of her skull. There was a specific area just inside her right eyebrow that did not feel normal. Closer examination revealed the faint impression of a scar, prompting her mother to recall that at the age of two Amy had fallen against a radiator. There had been lots of blood, a hospital visit and then the incident was forgotten.

Through the bones of the skull, what caught my attention at this particular point was a 'pull' or tension in the dura, the tough membrane which lines the skull and encloses the brain. This area

* All case studies in this book reflect genuine cases. Names and other circumstantial details have been changed to preserve patient confidentiality.

forms the housing of a region of the brain that manages some very primitive emotions, including violent urges. By 'cradling' the skull and exerting a very light pressure in a specific direction, using techniques practised over many years, I was able to release the pull of the dura and normalise the housing of this part of the brain. Amy's behaviour greatly improved following the treatment.

HISTORICAL HEAD TRAUMAS AND LONG-TERM MENTAL HEALTH PROBLEMS

News headlines these days tell the stories of many well-known football and rugby players developing early onset Alzheimer's following multiple head impacts during their sporting years. This is just one of the distressing long-term outcomes now being recognised as a consequence of repetitive head trauma. Mood disorders and other brain degenerative conditions are also involved.

There are more than 5 million rugby players worldwide, 1.6 million ice hockey players, 3 million field hockey players, 250 million football players, plus all the boxers, cricket players, winter sportsmen and women and others involved in impact sports. A proportion of this hugely significant number of sportsmen and women – and children – may be suffering needlessly with mood disorders at present or will suffer in the future as a consequence of head trauma. That head trauma may be a single strong blow or a low-grade repetitive trauma as in heading a football or being repeatedly punched.

As well as sportspeople there are estimated to be in America alone some 4.5 million people (adults and children) wearing teeth braces. This represents a low-grade insidious trauma on the skull and can create a similar scenario. Then there are those who have suffered blows to the head through car accidents, falls, attacks or just simply walking into a cupboard door!

MEMBRAIN DISORDER

'Membrain' is the term used in this book to describe the intimate relationship between the dural membrane and the brain itself. 'Membrain disorder', the topic of the first part of this book, means a physical condition which, once recognised, allows for a successful therapeutic approach to mental health problems arising from physical head trauma(s). The traumas to the head may be recent or historical. Membrain disorder can be caused by a head injury which, left untreated as in Amy's case, may in the shorter term cause mood disorders such as depression or anxiety and in the longer term lead to brain diseases such as dementia. Such a link has been established statistically in the case of rugby and football players and others who have suffered sport-related head traumas, but the nature of the link remains obscure to medical scientists. 'Membrain disorder' offers an explanation of that 'missing link' and a possible solution to the problem, which involves treating the environment of the brain.

THE ENVIRONMENT OF THE BRAIN

The brain and connected spinal cord sit in a flexible 'bag' (the dural membrane) and the bag sits in a more rigid 'box' (the skull). The brain, the bag and the box are all impacted in a head trauma, however slight that impact, and yet only the brain, up until now, has been considered worthy of medical attention. Yet it is the skull, the brain's housing, that directly receives every impact.

The dura mater is a tough, double-layered, tadpole-shaped membrane lining the skull and spinal canal. When the dura is disturbed by a problem in the skull, including a legacy of a past injury, the dura responds by changing its shape. A change in the shape of the dura affects the brain, in part through a distortion of the space in which the brain sits and in part due to the disruption of fluid circulation. Blood collects and leaves the skull via a complex venous sinus system that sits between the two layers of the dura.

Unimpeded exit of the blood is vital to prevent any backlog of fluids and build-up of congestion, like a motorway becoming clogged by a blocked motorway exit. The vital irrigation system of the brain relies heavily on the state of the dura. When irrigation is compromised, so is the vital supply of oxygen, nutrients and information to the brain and there is a build-up of elimination (waste) products that cannot find an efficient exit channel.[3]

The dura, the skull and the irrigation system of the brain together form the brain's environment. If the environment of the brain is disrupted, this will have consequences for the brain's behaviour and this can manifest as a mood disorder: a mental health issue. If the brain's environment is disrupted over a long period of time this can lead to a permanent degeneration of the brain tissue: a brain disease.

It is possible, following a head impact, to diagnose and treat membrain disorder via the dural membrane system so that the brain's housing returns to normal before any lasting damage is done. The treatment can have an immediate effect on mental health and bring long-term benefit to the overall health of the brain. Timely treatment of membrain disorder can both restore membrain health and prevent long-term damage. As seen in Amy's case, even the effects of a 'legacy' injury sustained years ago can be successfully addressed.

MEMBRAIN DISORDER IS JUST ONE AMONG OTHER CAUSES

Mental health problems are of many kinds and have many different origins, of which membrain disorder is only one. However, correctly recognising the origin, or origins, of a problem is vital in identifying the right treatment (as discussed in Part Two of this book). In Amy's case, the principal cause of her behavioural difficulties was a long-term tension or deformation in the dura. This was affecting Amy's brain and ultimately her ability to control her temper and violent urges. All of this stemmed from a forgotten and seemingly unimportant childhood injury to her skull that had left a physical legacy that was starting to show itself – and it was treatable. These physical legacies can start to make themselves noticed when the body is subjected to new stresses, perhaps unrelated to the original trauma. They can be physical (perhaps another blow to the head), emotional (maybe starting a new school, or stress at home) or a change to the body's chemistry. In Amy's case she had started going through puberty. This could have been the trigger.

A hands-on approach which addresses the dural membrane is not a cure-all. If there has been a head trauma that has passed through the protective skull and membrane system and directly damaged brain tissue then a hands-on therapeutic approach cannot offer a solution, certainly not immediately.

Moreover, many patients living with mental health issues, probably the majority, experience disturbed behaviour and feelings from causes other than head impacts. These include major emotional upheavals or challenging long-term health problems. For such patients the appropriate treatment might involve well-known 'talking therapies' from a psychotherapist, a clinical psychologist or a counsellor. These talking therapists may use specialist approaches such as CBT* or EMDR†. For those whose mental health problems are of familial origin this may be learned behaviour or have a genetic basis. Where there is an imbalance of vital chemicals in the brain, psychotropic drugs prescribed by a psychiatrist will be more helpful. Such patients are unlikely to respond to a mechanical hands-on approach looking to diagnose and treat membrane dysfunction as a cause. In short, membrain disorder is just one of many possible contributory factors that can lead to mental health issues, but I am writing this book because

* Cognitive Behavioural Therapy
† Eye Movement Desensitization and Reprocessing

it is a significant cause and it is unrecognised in current mental health diagnostics and almost invariably goes untreated.

THE AIM OF THIS BOOK

The primary aim of this book is to bring the concept of 'membrain health' and recognition of the condition termed 'membrain disorder' to the attention of patients, therapists, GPs, other medics and mental health professionals.

The 'medical model' prevalent in the medical and mental health professions does not consider the brain's housing – its physical environment – when considering psychological health. GPs, psychiatrists and other mental health practitioners are practised in identifying the social environmental factors of individuals with mental health problems – such as difficult relationships, money problems, housing issues and discrimination. There is also a great deal of research on the brain itself, but little attention to the physical *environment* of the brain.

'Membrain health' denotes a healthy physical environment of the brain: the brain housed comfortably inside the dural membrane, bathed and nourished via a healthy irrigation system. The brain is unchallenged by its environment.

Membrain disorder explains the straightforward physical process through which even minor trauma to the skull – if left untreated – can cause immediate or delayed mood disorders and potentially leave a physical legacy for the brain and its housing that can over time lead to serious brain disease. Diagnosis is based on a patient's history, observation of their head and face and palpation of the underlying membrane system.

Observation and palpation were the skill set of the previous generation of GPs but these tools have been largely discarded and replaced by technology. The problem is that palpation cannot be measured, only described. In the absence of an actual skull fracture, mechanical shifts and changes to the cranial bones and underlying dural membrane system do not show up as discrepancies on an X-Ray, MRI scan, CT scan, blood test, etc. To address membrain disorder, the skills of observation and palpation would need to be reinstated as valid diagnostic tools alongside the technological advances made in the orthodox medical world. Once diagnosed, membrain disorder can be successfully treated by a trained manual practitioner with the skills to restore membrain health.

COMPLEXITY AND MENTAL HEALTH: THE DIMENSIONAL MODEL

The second part of the book discusses mental health more broadly and encourages a different perspective from that prevailing in the current world of mental health diagnosis and care.

It is an approach to diagnosis and treatment of psychological illness built around an understanding of 'complexity' – an understanding embraced in other fields such as climate change and pollution management. The approach to diagnosis set out in Part Two bears some relationship to the influential 'biopsychosocial' model introduced by George Engel in his article "The Need for a New Medical Model".[4]

Writing at a time when the thoughts, emotions and social circumstances of a patient were increasingly being dismissed by the medical profession as utterly irrelevant to disease, Engel called for a holistic 'systems theory' approach to life-processes in which the biological *and* psychological *and* social aspects of illness are taken seriously and understood as different levels operating together within a whole system. The system includes molecules, cells and organs, the whole organism (the human being), and society, or the biosphere. As an example, a diagnosis of cancer is not 'just' identification of a physical disease to be resolved by drugs or surgery. The diagnosis – and the treatment process – may have a profound impact on the patient's own thoughts and feelings and affect family and work colleagues, practically and emotionally. These are very real aspects of cancer. Moreover, social factors such as poor housing, unhealthy diet and pollution are known to increase rates of cancer, regardless of a person's individual genetic inheritance. Hence, 'cancer' cannot be thought of simply as a biomedical issue within a patient's body.

Much discussion in the first part of this book centres around the brain and its environment, but the brain represents just one dimension of a very complex human social and biological system. In this book that system is pictured as six linked 'dimensions', ranging from the microscopic realm of chemical reactions within our cells to the large-scale social dimension in which we live our lives (the six dimensions are explained in chapter 10). A mental health issue can originate in any one (or sometimes more than one) of these dimensions, and practitioners need to know the source of the problem in order to treat it effectively.

Like many practitioners today, I share Engel's holistic view of illness,[5] but the emphasis in this book is specifically on mental health, and on identifying the levels or dimensions at which mental health issues *originate and can be treated* in each patient's case.

This perspective on mental health diagnosis and care takes the emphasis away from labelling a condition based on a patient's display of *symptoms* and focuses on the *origin* of a patient's mental health problems. The common diagnosis of 'depression', for example, is based on a collection of familiar symptoms but it can originate from any of the six different dimensions discussed in the book. A patient may be depressed because they lack certain chemicals in the brain and this is an inherited family trait (biomolecular dimension). They may be depressed because of a fall causing a head injury (brain dimension). Or they may be going through a hideous divorce and this is the cause of depression (whole person dimension). These are all very different origins, but the label 'depression' is shared by all because the symptoms are similar. This easily leads to the same treatment being prescribed for conditions that, below the surface, are very different. This book will argue that it is not the label but the dimension of origin of an individual's mental health issue that is crucial when carrying out a diagnosis and deciding how best to help that individual patient.

THE READER

Mind & Membrain is written for both the general reader and health practitioners (GPs, clinicians, manual and talking therapists). I hope it will be of interest to the sports world and offer some direction in which to channel their investigations into head trauma and its distressing outcomes. It introduces a new concept to one and all.

It may be that the reader is looking for a practical solution to a specific mental health problem either personally or for someone they know and Part One of the book provides all the information required to decide whether membrain disorder could be relevant in a particular case.

The wider perspective on mental health offered in Part Two of the book offers patients and health practitioners an alternative understanding of the dimensional origin(s) of a mental health problem, with complexity in mind. This provides a much-needed metaphorical 'road map' (see Appendix) to determine which type of therapy among the many available could be most effective and why.

The beginnings of both Part One and Part Two are necessarily quite technical but if the reader can push through these technical parts they will access the detailed anonymised case histories of patients who have been diagnosed and treated. These present living examples of the diagnosis and treatment of membrain disorder and the further dimensional diagnosis of mental health problems.

There is a Glossary at the end of the book which explains terms which may be unfamiliar to non-specialist readers.

THE WRITER

Jo Wildy draws on more than thirty years of clinical experience as an osteopath practising in the cranial field with a specialism in treating patients with mental health problems. She has a clinical practice in the UK and in addition has taught osteopathy in the cranial field for over 20 years, predominantly in northern Europe where her students are fully qualified physiotherapists and medical doctors enrolled on a six-year masters programme in osteopathy.

In the UK osteopathy sits on the outside of the orthodox system in contrast with Northern Europe and other places where it is far more integrated. It takes time and it takes practice but anyone in the medical field – if he or she is inclined to do so – can learn to feel ('palpate') and treat the head, including successfully treating membrain disorder.

Alongside her clinical and teaching experience, Jo Wildy has explored the science around natural laws, studying complexity theory as applied to biological systems and in particular the human being. This involves a thorough understanding of evolutionary processes as well as the development of the human embryo from fertilized egg to birth. Chronology (the sequence of events in time) becomes an important factor when considering how biological systems form and maintain themselves and their interdependence. This approach offers a new understanding of health and disease.

In her years of study and professional practice Jo Wildy has come to recognise that any problem with the environment or housing of an organ or system within the body is very real and potentially serious for the system concerned, whether this is the brain, the digestive or respiratory system or any other part of the body. Abnormal housing will affect the adaptive behaviour of that organ or system as it struggles to maintain itself and this can produce symptoms even though the physical structure of the organ or system remains unaltered. In the case of the brain, the symptom may, for example, be a mood disorder.

If the abnormal housing persists long-term, the organ or system under prolonged stress will change its structure and it is at this stage that irreversible changes will take place. In the case of the brain this may be a neurodegenerative disorder involving physical changes to the brain that can take a variety of forms such as Parkinson's, Alzheimer's, or Chronic Traumatic Encephalopathy (CTE), amongst others. One knock to the skull from heading a football or colliding with another player can disturb the brain's environment. Repeated knocks will almost certainly do so.

PREVENTION IS BETTER THAN CURE

Statistical studies reveal a clear link between repeated sporting head trauma and early onset dementia, but the only solution offered seems to be to limit further and further the possibility of head impacts by banning heading the ball in football or outlawing contact rugby for youngsters. Even with these highly unpopular measures in place, head injuries will always occur. They can happen to anyone at any age for other reasons – a difficult birth, an accident or an assault, even surgical or dental treatment.

In all cases of known head trauma, an effective preventive approach would be to examine the subject for possible membrain disorder and, if this is diagnosed, help the brain's housing to return to normal through manual therapy. The treatment is a gentle and effective treatment, with the aim of restoring membrain health.

Everything in this book is based on straightforward ideas and clinical experience. There is no magical thinking, just as there are no magical cures, just a different way of thinking about mental health, presented here to be further explored by both patients and professionals.

PART ONE

MEMBRAIN DISORDER

ONE

THE SKULL IS A LIVING STRUCTURE

THE SKULL

It is a common assumption that the skull is a fixed, inert and solid bony structure. It 'protects' the brain, most people imagine, rather like a builder's hard hat. To understand the concept of the skull as part of the brain's living environment, an environment that can change, this assumption needs a radical rethink and a re-introduction to the skull and to its neglected but crucially important underlying membrane system, the dura.

A skull (medical name, cranium) is composed of three main bony parts: a *cranial vault*, a *cranial base* and a *face* (figure 1). The three main parts (vault, base and face) develop together from the very start of life and sit in a positional relationship with one another – rather like children living in the same house who grow together and are affected by one another.

Each of the three parts is in turn made up of smaller bones – there are twenty-two in all (figure 2). The twenty-two smaller bones connect together in a complex and engineered way. Over the decades there will be some fusion (merging) between individual bones in some places, but in many areas the parts remain separate

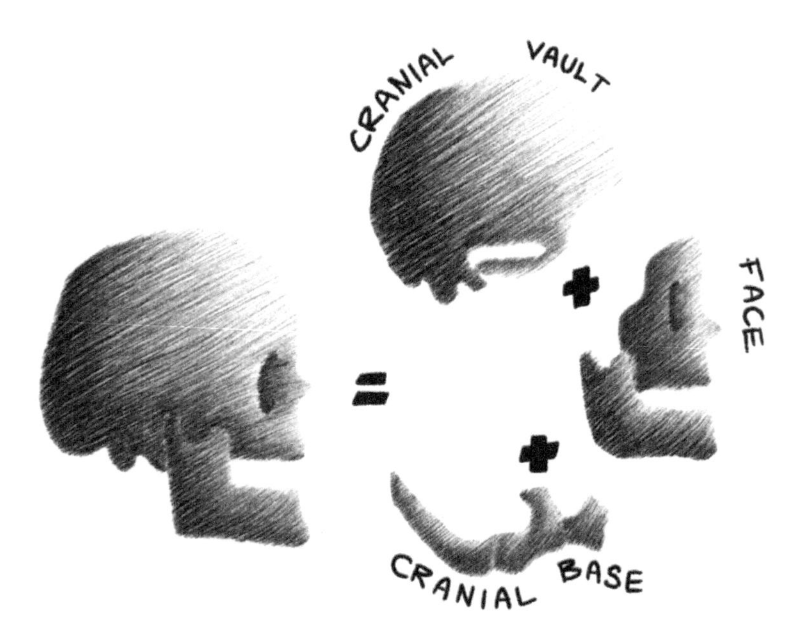

Figure 1. The cranium is made up of three main parts – the vault, the base, and the face.

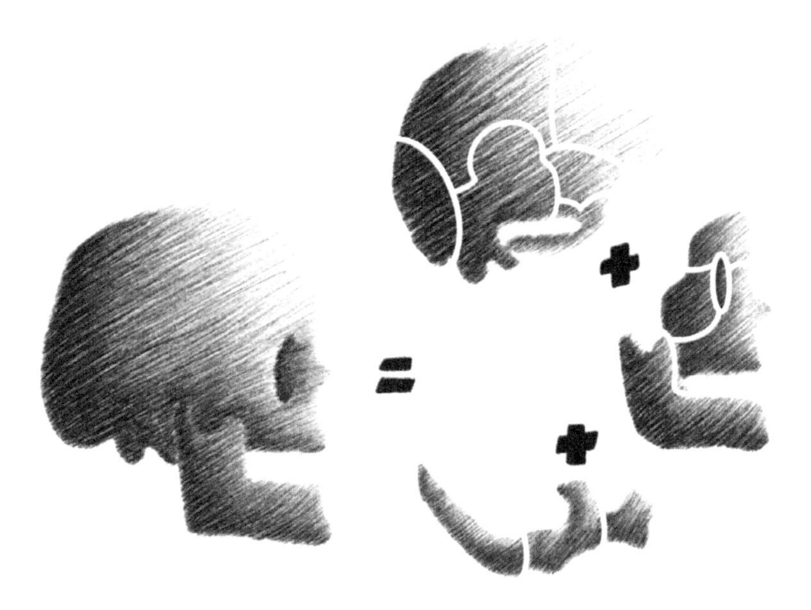

Figure 2. The three main parts of the cranium comprise 22 individual bones.

– rather like a completed jigsaw puzzle, where the pieces are kept in place due to their shape but are not glued together.

One way to visualise the whole bony skull is indeed as a three-dimensional jigsaw puzzle, perhaps one portraying a globe of the world. If any of the twenty-two bones of the skull are disturbed in their relationships to neighbouring bones, this upsets the biomechanics of that area of the skull and possibly the whole of the skull (figure 3).

If at any point in a person's life there is a change in the way the parts of the skull fit together (for example at different stages of growth, or if a part of the skull is injured) there will have to be an adaptation around that change. Bone is a strong, dense structure but it is not a lifeless material like plastic or metal. It is a living substance; it is resilient. This is easily seen when, say, a bone in the arm is fractured. The bone will react and the damaged parts will fuse back together. When the damage is not visible, for example a subtle change in positional relationships as shown in figure 3B, as is so often true of knocks to the head, the bones of the skull will nonetheless have reacted and tried to adapt to the change – but how?

THE DURA

Underneath the skull is a strong membrane called the *dura mater* (Latin for 'tough mother', which in turn is a translation from an Arabic medical term meaning 'tough mother of the brain' – a very good description!)*

As shown in figure 4, the dura is a vertical, tadpole-shaped bag made of a strong, flexible double membrane. At certain places within the skull this double membrane separates to create a midline vertical divider and two horizontal dividers which divide

* Anatomically speaking, there are three layers of membrane that surround the brain, one inside the other. The outer one (just inside the skull) is the 'tough mother', the dura mater. Within that is the arachnoid mater and within that the pia mater. In this book 'dura' always refers to the dura mater.

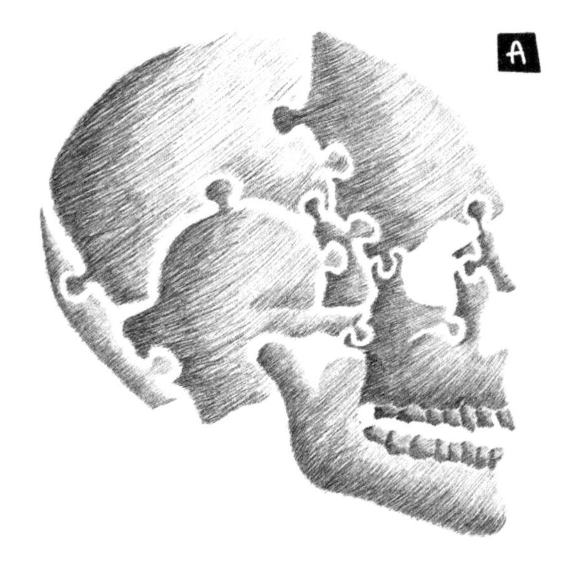

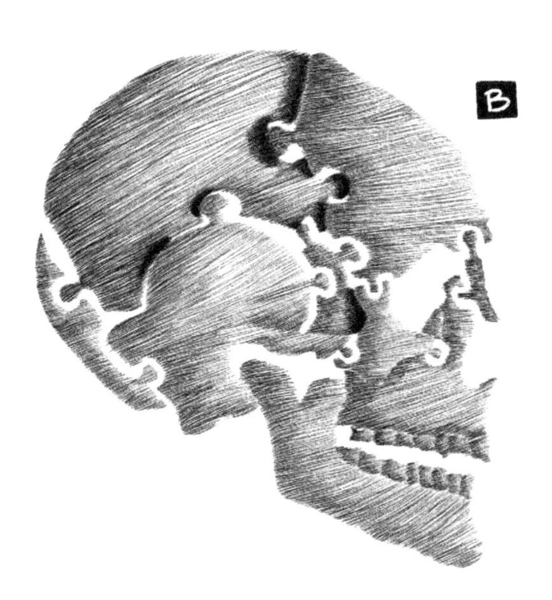

Figure 3. The three-dimensional jigsaw puzzle – a visual analogy of the skull. (A) Normal relationships of the parts. (B) Altered relationships of the parts.

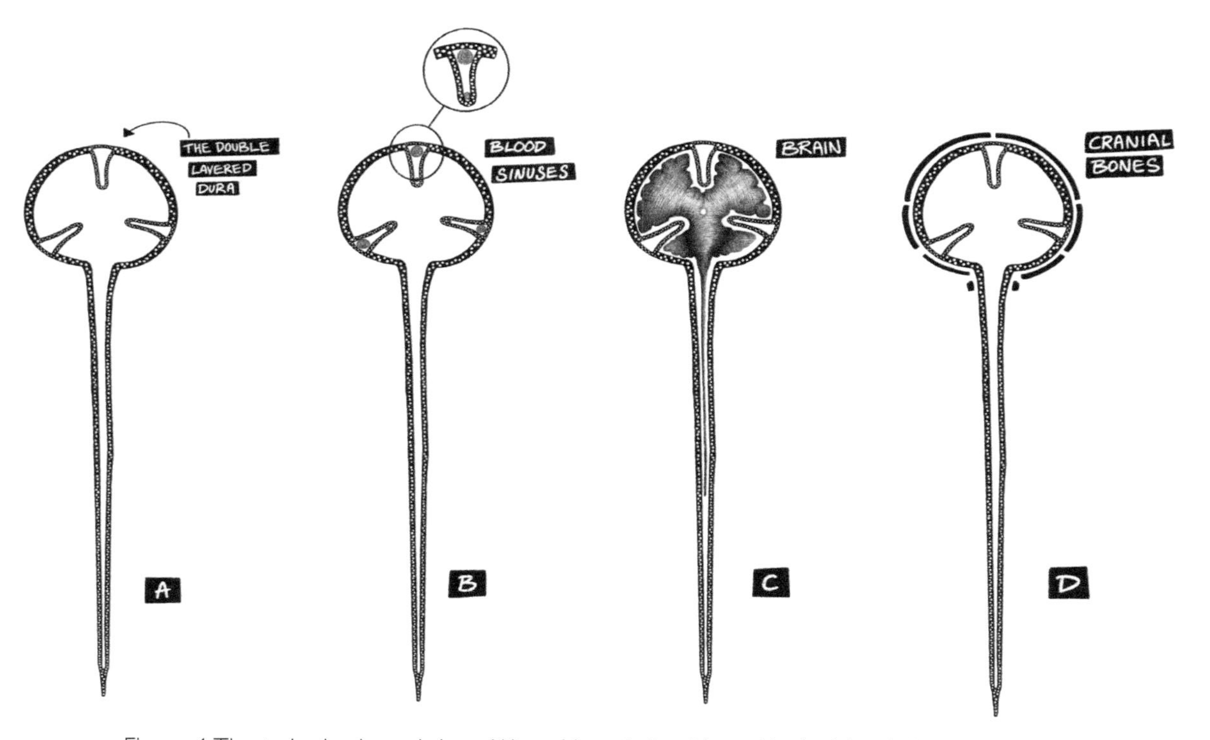

Figure 4. The tadpole-shaped dura (A) and its relationships with the blood sinus system (B), the brain (C), and the cranial bones (D).

the cranial cavity into compartments: left and right, top and bottom (A).[6] Sitting between the two layers of the dura, within the dividers, is the venous sinus system responsible for the effective drainage of blood from the confined space of the cranial cavity back towards the heart (B).

The head of the tadpole-like dura surrounds the brain while the long tail encloses the spinal cord (the rope of nerves inside the spine stretching from the brain all the way down to the lower back). In short, the entire central nervous system (brain and spinal cord) is enclosed in the tadpole-shaped dura bag (C). Together they constitute the membrain. At the top (the head of the tadpole) the dura has attachments to specific points on the inside of the skull. At the other end (the tail of the tadpole) the dura has connections to the pelvis and coccyx (D).

If there is a problem in the skull (such as a bang on the head) which makes a change, however tiny, to the relationship between the bones of the skull, the dura will very cleverly alter its tadpole shape, creating what can be described as a pull or pulls onto those points of attachment. In effect, the dura is shifting the bones of the skull around to get them back to normal. It is trying to auto-correct any altered relationship between the three main bony parts of the skull, or between the twenty-two individual smaller bones.

The dura is an alert and reactive membrane system with a rich nerve supply and capable of exerting a surprisingly strong influence on the bones of the skull.

The dura (figure 5) is a dynamic structure that shifts between a short fat and a long narrow shape (B & C). A problem arises when it becomes fixed in either extreme such that it cannot be adaptive. In someone experiencing inertia it is common to find the dura unable to release out of the short fat shape (B). In the classic 'fight or flight' response to a perceived threat or fright the dura becomes long and narrow. If the dura gets stuck in this *physical* state it will be difficult for an individual to release themselves from their agitated *mental*

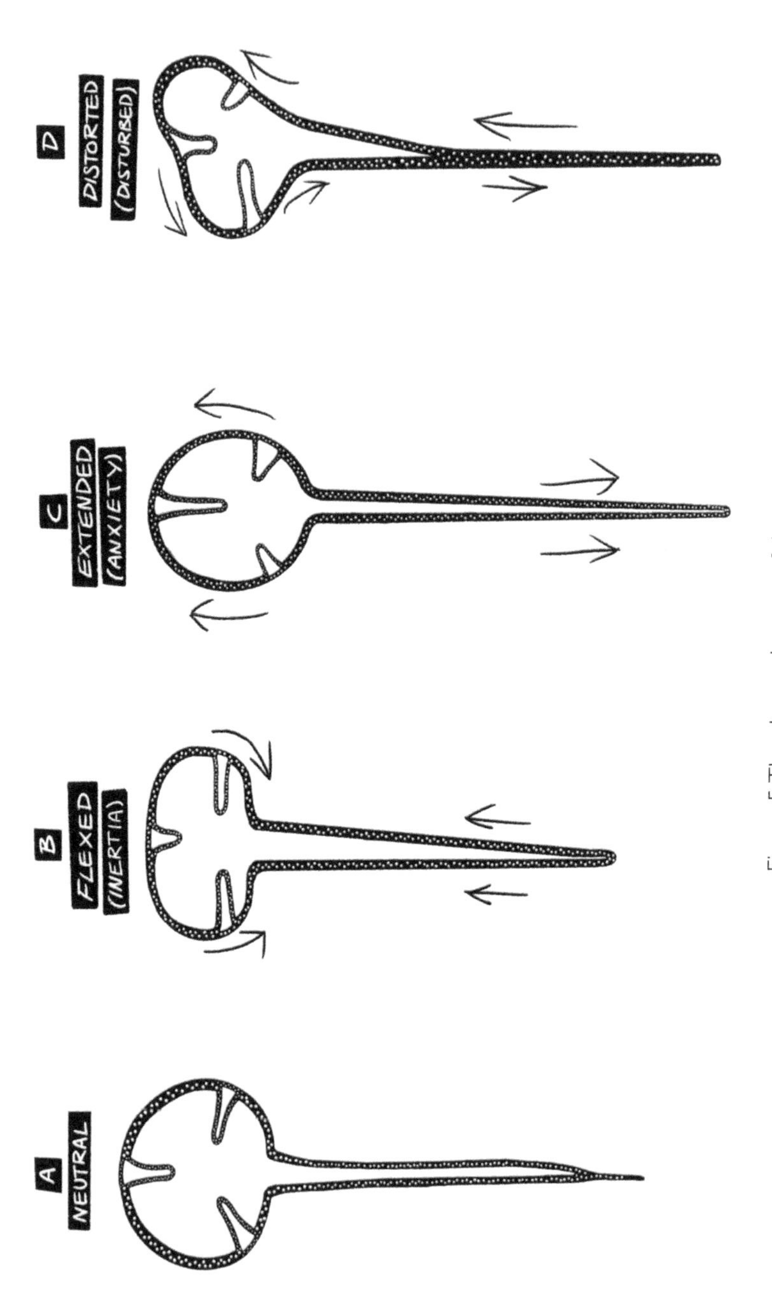

Figure 5. The shape changes of the dura.

state (C). As former international rugby player Kieran Bracken describes it: "You know if someone comes round a corner at you and shouts: 'Boo!' you'd get that rush of adrenaline? That was happening to me on a minute-by-minute basis. And I couldn't stop it."[7]

Alternatively the dura's tadpole shape becomes what can be described as 'distorted' (D) when there is a mismatch between the different main parts of the skull (the face, cranial base and cranial vault) or between the smaller individual bones of the skull. This is a mechanical problem and the dura is reacting to it in order to self-correct. If the distorted shape is persistent and unable to self-correct then the housing and irrigation of the brain area is compromised. Membrain health is lost. This in turn can affect thinking, emotions and behaviour.

(It is possible for the reader to pull their whole body into a shape that mirrors these four forms and pay attention to the instant effect it has on how they 'feel'. Then one can imagine being 'stuck' in that state, unable to release from it – and how that might make someone feel over time.)

DIAGNOSIS AND TREATMENT VIA THE DURA

It is through this enterprising dural membrane system that it is possible to diagnose and treat the skull and thus influence the living environment of the brain. A skilled manual practitioner trained in the cranial field is able to diagnose a 'mechanical' problem in the skull where there is a mismatch in the positional relationships of its twenty-two parts via the response of the underlying membrane system as it attempts to self-correct. The dura 'wants' to restore the skull to its proper form.

The practitioner treats the patient by supporting the dura, offering a fulcrum or an extra impetus to what is already happening. The technique involves 'cradling' the skull in a particular position, a very light contact on the skull and a strong fulcrum, located back along the practitioner's arms as far as the elbows. The approach works by interacting with the dura, supporting what it is already trying to do and sometimes adding a little extra. It is literally giving the dura a helping hand. If successful, then a change occurs. The dura, with that extra help, manages to resolve the problem and normal relationships among the bones of the skull are re-established. Left untreated, if the dura is unable to restore order to the skull, the dura's capacity to cope with further problems is diminished. It can become fatigued, agitated or congested. Even a few knocks to the head at different stages of life can have a cumulative effect, so the repetitive head injuries typical of sports such as football or rugby are particularly dangerous.

In manual therapy, every individual case and its treatment is different and it is difficult to put in words exactly how work on the dura-skull relationship is managed, just as it would be difficult to put in words exactly how one plays a particular piece of music on a particular instrument. Treating a deformation of the skull through the dura is a very specific, practical skill which is 'learned' by the hands as much as the mind. It is impossible to predict precisely what effect a treatment on the skull and membrane system will have on the brain, much as it is difficult to predict exactly how a piece of music will affect the person listening to it. The practitioner is not treating the brain directly. How the brain responds to its environment being restored to normal is entirely up to nature. In nature, systems are generally able to maintain themselves and behave normally in unchallenging environments.

If the practitioner is successful, the housing of the brain will return to normal and this has a beneficial effect on the behaviour of the brain. Because the brain manages thoughts and emotions as well as physical processes, psychological symptoms will ease and even disappear altogether – always assuming that abnormal housing – membrain disorder – was a contributing factor to the patient's condition.

The concept of 'housing' of the brain is key here, because the skull and dura and the fluids they contain constitute the living environment of the brain. As explained earlier, the environment of any organ or system affects the behaviour of that system. The next chapter will examine that process in more detail.

TWO

'SICK BUILDING SYNDROME'

IT IS THE STATE OF THE BUILDING THAT CAUSES ITS OCCUPANTS TO SUFFER

From late 2020 onwards, headline news reports have been appearing of football and rugby players campaigning for recognition of the link between youthful contact sports, mood disorders and serious brain diseases in later life. There is overwhelming evidence that footballers are over three times more likely than the rest of the population to suffer from degenerative brain diseases.[8] Rugby players report a high incidence of depression – way above the national average.[9] Much the same applies to boxers, cricket and hockey players, those who compete in bobsleigh and the luge and other sports with a risk of head impacts – and the problem affects both men and women.[10]

THE MISSING LINK

Despite the statistics, scientists are still seeking to understand what the physical link is between knocks to the head in one's youth and irreversible brain disease years later (leaving room for the sports authorities and their insurers to question the nature of the link and where their responsibility lies).[11,12] Least of all does anyone seem to understand what preventive or corrective action would eliminate the risks. But even if contact sports were banned the problem would still exist – head injuries can be caused in many ways. There are no explanations, no ideas of what can be done to remedy things – except perhaps the imposition of ever more health and safety precautions.

'THE KILLER INSIDE: THE MIND OF AARON HERNANDEZ'

There is a Netflix series 'The Killer Inside: The Mind of Aaron Hernandez' which documents the life of a young American sportsman. Aaron Hernandez had been one of the top American football players before his suicide in prison in 2017. He was 27 years old. He had played football for his high school and had already achieved national recognition as an outstanding athlete before going professional. Yet during his short life he was involved in a number of violent episodes, had numerous run-ins with the law and in 2015 was imprisoned for murder. It was only after his suicide in prison that anyone thought to investigate his brain, despite the already known association of brain disease, moods and altered behaviour in athletes subject to repeated head injury.

Anyone watching the Netflix footage of Hernandez playing will see his head get battered, battered and then battered again. When the authorities did a brain autopsy on Hernandez subsequent to his death they found a disease common enough to have by now its own medical name: Chronic Traumatic Encephalopathy or CTE. CTE is a degenerative brain disease found in athletes and others with a history of repetitive head trauma.[13] Early symptoms of CTE usually appear in a patient's late twenties or thirties and affect both mood and behaviour. Some common symptoms include impulse control problems, aggression, depression, and paranoia. Aaron Hernandez' brain was said to be the worst case the pathologists had seen in someone so young (figure 6).

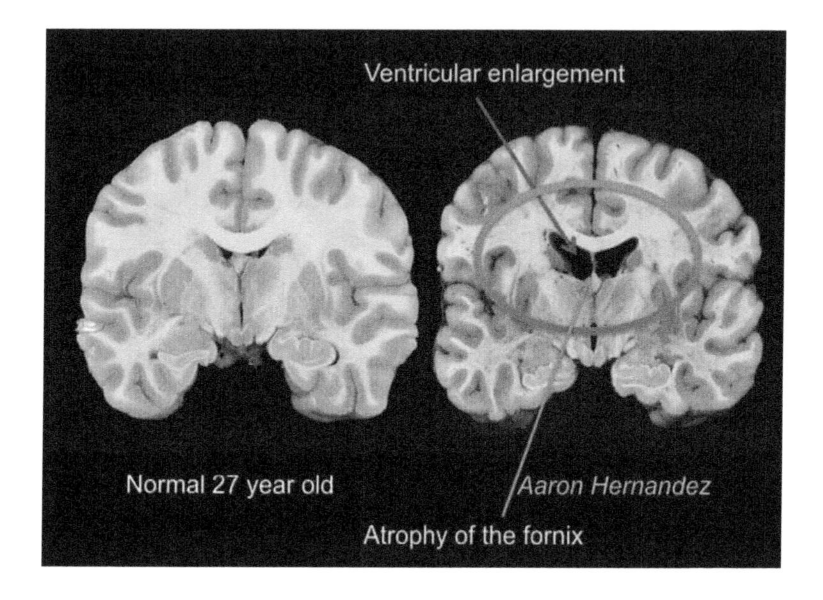

Figure 6. Cross section of a normal brain (left) and that of Aaron Hernandez at the time of his death (right). Image: Dr Ann McKee, Boston University School of Medicine.

It is important to note the precise terms used in the scientific literature about CTE. The authors will refer to 'brain trauma' or 'traumatic brain injury' (TBI) as being the cause of the behavioural and mood changes, but this is just an assumption. These athletes have been subjected to repetitive *head* injury. The general assumption is that any bang on the head must travel through and damage the brain tissue then and there. Yet it is the skull, the outer casing, that most obviously takes the beating. What is never considered is whether CTE might be caused by injuries to the *housing* of the brain – the skull – and that it is the skull injury leading to membrain disorder that has an influence on the brain – not immediately but over time.

Membrain disorder may cause mood disorders and behavioural problems in the shorter term. Over a longer period it may lead to the gradual changes of degenerative brain diseases recorded in those statistical surveys in boxers, footballers, and others (including homeless people) shown to have a high incidence of head injuries.

SICK BUILDING SYNDROME – AN ANALOGY

Imagine an office block that has seen better days. The windows are small and not designed to open, so no fresh air and very little natural light comes into the office. The ventilation system controls the temperature poorly; it is either too cold or too hot and the same air is recirculated. The sewage system gets blocked periodically leading to unwanted smells. The occupants of that building, the work force, will not thrive over time. Some members of the work force may become physically sick or mentally unwell. The work force becomes depleted. This is what is known as 'Sick Building Syndrome'.[14,15] "Over time" is very relevant here

Sick building syndrome can be described as an 'outside-inside' phenomenon. The health or behaviour of any system, wherever one looks, at whatever level one looks, is dependent to a very large extent on its environment. The system is the 'inside' and sits within its environment – the 'outside' – but in fact the two are intricately linked. A system will always respond to its environment and that response can be described as a *behaviour*.

For example, a group of water molecules will behave as ice, water, or steam, dependent entirely on the temperature and pressure of their environment. A body of water will behave as a tidal stream in response to gravitational pulls from the moon and the sun. The behaviour of a sunflower is to turn its head to follow the light and warmth of the sun as it moves from East to West through the day.

Sick Building Syndrome facilitates an understanding of how the behaviour of the brain can be adversely influenced by its environment. The brain is like the office staff, who need to be fit and alert to coordinate and perform all sorts of complicated activities properly (their normal behaviour). The protective housing of the brain is the building. The irrigation of the brain – the provision of nutrients and oxygen via the blood supply and the removal of used products to and from the brain – is equivalent to the lighting, ventilation and plumbing system of the building. When the environment is poor, the workers' behaviour is adversely affected. The behaviour of the brain, just like the behaviour of the office staff, changes according to its environmental conditions over time – as does any system. Eventually the brain will not just change its behaviour but become depleted.

THE ENVIRONMENT OF THE BRAIN

The dura, the bony parts of the skull, and fluids flowing into, through and back out of the cranium constitute the physical environment of the brain. The brain effectively sits in a bag and the bag sits in a box (figure 7). If any of this environment is disturbed, the brain will, sooner or later, be disturbed too.

W. G. Sutherland, the founding father of osteopathy in the cranial field, discovered over a century ago through self-experimentation – applying constant pressure to different parts of his own skull – that if the mechanics of the skull are subject to a physical strain then psychological distress can be an outcome.

What WGS clearly understood is that the condition of the skull can have a huge influence on the behaviour of the brain and this affects the psychological health of an individual. This knowledge is shared by all those who have subsequently trained and worked in the cranial field but so far the phenomenon hasn't been given a name. The new term 'membrain disorder' used in this book describes a malfunctioning of the brain due to disruption of its environment. A malfunctioning of the brain can directly affect actions, thoughts and feelings.

Membrain disorder is then the 'missing' physical link behind the statistics which show that those prone to repeated low-grade injuries or single heavy impacts to the skull have an increased likelihood of developing behavioural problems, mood disorders and early onset of degenerative brain disease.

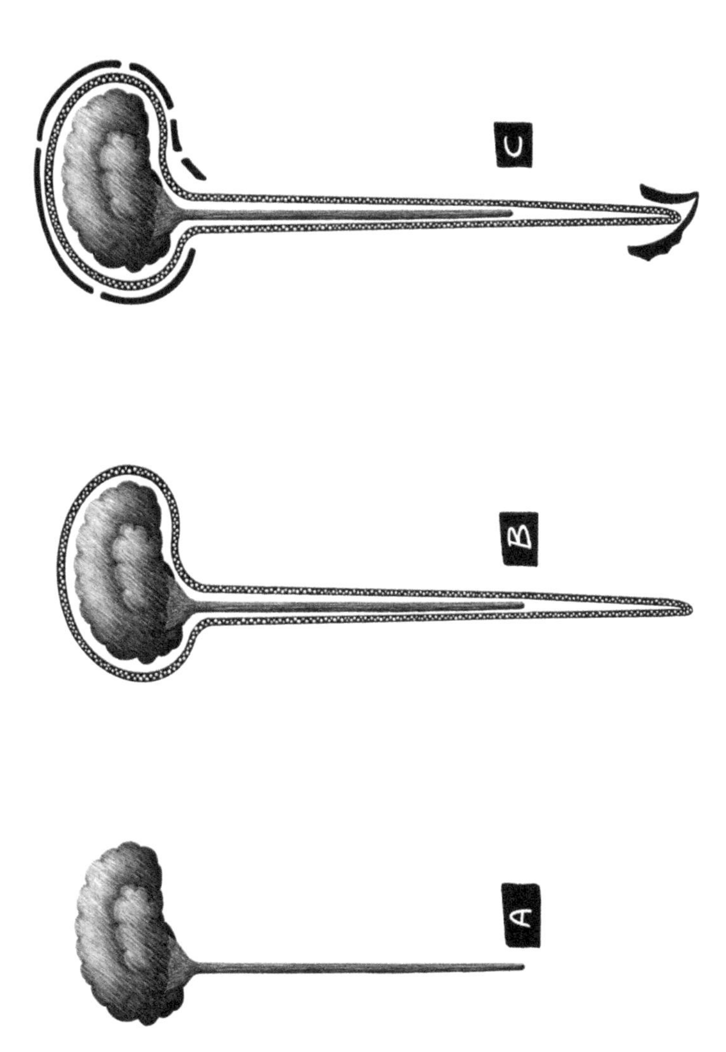

Figure 7. The Brain (A) in a Bag (B) in a Box (C).

BRAIN TRAUMA VERSUS MEMBRAIN DISORDER

Membrain disorder – a disturbance of the housing of the brain – has to be clearly distinguished from brain trauma where there is direct injury to the brain itself.

Direct brain injury – brain trauma – occurs when the skull is fractured and the underlying brain tissue is directly damaged. Head injury or head shaking too can cause bleeding in or around the brain even without fracturing the skull. The extra pressure of the blood, or deprivation of blood supply to an area of the brain, will in these cases very shortly cause direct brain damage. Such events will show up on a brain scan.

Then there is concussion, a common but loosely defined term to describe an injury to the brain even though in most cases no visible damage shows up on a brain scan. Mild concussion may mean 'seeing stars' and temporary disorientation but it may take the form of full-blown concussion where the person whose skull has taken a blow will suffer a loss of consciousness soon after the injury. This can lead on to a condition called 'post-concussion syndrome' where patients can take months or even years for their brain to recover from such an incident. They suffer headaches or hallucinations, an inability to concentrate, feel extremely tired and find computer and TV screens almost intolerable. The condition can be extremely debilitating and because the injury has impacted the brain directly there is a limit to how much a manual therapist can help, at least initially. Patients with a direct brain trauma may need both emergency medical treatment and time and rest for their brain to recover. In all such scenarios the head trauma has clearly had a direct and immediate impact on the brain.

A manual therapist cannot treat the brain directly – only its environment, the skull and dura. Once the brain has had time to recover from a direct brain injury it is worth examining the housing of the brain. The whole head, not just the brain, was subject to the trauma and it may be that the container of the brain, the skull, was also affected and that a legacy of that injury persists. If such a physical legacy persists it should be treated using a manual intervention. This can lead to a fuller recovery in the long term. There are a number of published case history studies describing the successful osteopathic treatment of patients with post-concussion syndrome, with various explanations for the efficacy of such an intervention.[16,17,18]

AN INVISIBLE LEGACY

Far more common than a diagnosed brain injury are the many head traumas that involve no visible structural damage to the skull or the brain. There is no skull fracture, no concussion, or the concussion is measured as mild and these cases are dismissed as insignificant. There are also those serial bangs to the head suffered by contact sports people. Case studies in this book show that in some of such cases (not all) a physical legacy of such an injury will remain, affecting the bony skull, the underlying dura and the irrigation system of the brain – in other words, membrain disorder. These are legacies that are not going to be picked up by X-Ray or MRI scan. They can however be picked up by palpation. They may have an immediate effect in the form of mood disorders such as depression, anxiety and OCD[19] but they are also legacies that, left undiagnosed and untreated, exert a different influence over time, sometimes over years or decades – namely causing a structural change to the brain tissue: a brain pathology such as CTE or forms of dementia.

A scientific study in 2018 compared the MRI scans of the brains of a number of recently retired contact sportsmen who were complaining of 'impaired executive function' (put simply, an inability to concentrate) with the scans of a control group of non-sportsmen of similar age.[20] The MRIs showed no significant differences, no signs of early changes to the soft brain tissue itself, in either group, despite the fact that only the retired sportsmen were complaining of psychological symptoms and were more anxious and more likely to report unusual thoughts and experiences. The paper's conclusion was that their mental health problems did not stem from sports brain injuries. However, no alternative cause was identified. By 2020, the statistical evidence for a link between sports head impacts and mental health problems had become front-page news.

Membrain disorder can provide the missing explanation for altered behaviour without observable changes to the brain tissue. It is significant that effects over time (sometimes decades) were not considered in the 2018 research paper. Other research offers preliminary evidence that depression precedes cognitive changes and this, should it be confirmed, would correlate with the membrain health concept.[21] Sportspeople could then be directed towards the appropriate treatment at an early stage. This would be a preventive approach, one which acknowledged that head impacts are inevitable but serious mental health consequences are not. As soon as players became aware of psychological problems possibly associated with contact sports injuries, their best course of action would be to seek out a manual therapist trained in the cranial field, not only to help with their current psychological issues but, crucially, to prevent even more serious longer-term diseases including dementia from developing. Regular checks of all members of a contact sports team, perhaps at the end of each season, would also provide a preventive measure.

Holly

Holly was an outstanding sportswoman, a netball player performing at the very top of her game. During a tightly-contested international match she collided with another player. An ambulance was called and Holly was rushed to A&E. A diagnosis of concussion was made and Holly was sent home from hospital to rest.

Holly did rest for several frustrating months following a

further diagnosis of post-concussion syndrome. She was seeing a physiotherapist for continuing pain in her neck and was taking anti-depressants when she first came to see me. "I was hoping you could help with the headaches I keep getting," she told me. "My friend recommended osteopathy. I am just so fed up with how long it is taking to get back to normal. I am really hoping to be at my best for the team selection trials for next season."

Holly had certainly suffered some sort of brain trauma but enough time had passed to allow for natural healing and I diagnosed Holly as suffering also with membrain disorder. She was ready for some manual treatment to help not only her headaches, but *also* her mental state *and* her neck pain. The distorted dural membrane system that was so clearly palpable was contributing to all those symptoms. I started to treat Holly and we were making steady progress when Holly was unexpectedly taken out of my care. My experience with professional athletes is that often they do not control who treats them – instead, the professional bodies and the coaches decide. The coaches – and indeed the athletes – want a fast return to training, so if a therapist doesn't deliver instant results, another therapist is summoned. Holly was not however a 'quick fix'.

There are many like Holly out there, suffering from a whole range of different symptoms caused by a skull impact: pain and hypersensitivity, poor attention, emotional problems, disturbed sleep, the list goes on. Many are being medicated unnecessarily, suffering for far longer than necessary and – as the statistics show – at serious risk of long-term consequences. As things stand at present, a diagnosis of membrain disorder is not even considered. Moreover, the method of diagnosis required (palpation) and the means of treatment (described in chapter 6) are specialised skills not currently taught in any medical school.

Very little of what is discussed about membrain disorder in this book is evaluated in published scientific studies, for the very simple fact that the mental health implications of a disorder of the brain's housing – despite being made known more than a century ago through WGS's experiments in applying pressure to his own skull – have been entirely overlooked. The idea is simply absent from global consciousness, so the relevant questions have never been asked.

It is very difficult to insist to Holly that she needs to return to check that the legacy of the head trauma has fully resolved, that she may still have membrain disorder without a formal recognition of such a condition and scientific evidence to back it up.

A NEW CONCEPT

Putting forward a concept that challenges medical orthodoxy implies that there is something important that medical science doesn't know. The advance of science often depends on replacing previous 'established' ideas with new ones, which can, understandably, expect to be met with scepticism. On the other hand, new ideas should not be rejected only because they differ from orthodoxy. In this case the current understanding that the skull and underlying membrane system are inert structures unworthy of attention needs a radical rethink. The concept of membrain disorder offers a simple physical explanation based on the clinical experience of those trained to observe, *palpate* and treat heads and faces. Clinicians with such capabilities are extraordinarily rare. Most clinicians would not think why they could possibly want to palpate a head. It will be new to medical scientists, but the knowledge on which it is based can be acquired by anyone trained in the skills to diagnose and treat membrain disorder. The difficulty at present is that those skills are not taught in medical school and no significant research has been conducted on the role of the skull and dura in regard to brain function and mental health.

Gaps like this exist in 'orthodox' medical knowledge because until a condition such as membrain disorder is officially recognised and labelled, that condition might as well not exist and no treatment will be proposed. And unless a drug or other treatment has been scientifically researched and found effective, then it is not accepted as a 'genuine' treatment. This means that if the medical and mental health establishment decides not to pursue scientific investigation into a particular concept or a particular treatment it is regarded as invalid. Even if it works in practice it will remain by default 'unscientific'. Drug companies, who fund the vast majority of research, are by definition hostile to treatments that are effective and don't involve drugs.

To establish some investigative trials is the next step. Meanwhile, clinical experience can provide its own form of evidence through case-study accounts of the diagnosis and treatment of membrain disorder.

THREE

THE 'BUILDING'

Freddie

I had been qualified for six years and only recently started my own osteopathic practice when I received a call from a deeply troubled mother. "My seventeen-year-old son has been diagnosed as schizophrenic," she faltered, then continued "I have heard about osteopathy and just wondered if you could look at Freddie's head." I could hear the desperation in her voice.

Schizophrenia, along with psychosis, is a particular kind of psychological distress that is distinct from depression, OCD or anxiety. These patients suffer a loss of contact with our shared reality. This might involve seeing or hearing things that other people cannot see or hear (termed hallucinations) or believing that things are happening in a way that – so far as others can tell – they are not (termed delusions). Dealing with these issues is beyond my personal remit simply because a clinical intervention at this level of suffering requires a collegiate approach in a supportive environment available twenty-four hours a day, whereas I am a sole practitioner. It is not because I think that a manual intervention to treat membrain disorder will not help. In cases where membrain disorder is involved, I believe it could certainly help. I said "No" to seeing her son and apologetically explained my reluctance and my reasons. Regardless, she insisted: "Could you just take a look at him?"

This was a very long time ago. With his mother's and Freddie's permission, I got a chance just to put my hands on his head, albeit fleetingly. This was enough to tell me that, in an ideal world, in better circumstances, perhaps in a mental health team setting and where Freddie was under constant supervision, I would have wanted to play a part in the treatment of this young man – because I could have helped him.

PLAGIOCEPHALY

Just looking at Freddie across the desk, it was possible to observe that he had a visible plagiocephaly. Plagiocephaly is the medical term for an asymmetrical skull. Perfect symmetry rarely exists in nature, including in the human form, but there are degrees of asymmetry. Plagiocephaly in simple terms means a distorted skull. Such a condition is often, but not always, visible in the face, most notably a deviated jaw, and differently set or shaped eyes. The ears are often offset to one another and the cranial vault would be odd shaped, if not hidden by hair. Such features are visible to the trained eye but go unnoticed by most people.

It is important at this point to understand that plagiocephaly does not mean that someone will have mental health problems. Asymmetry is entirely natural and the body can adjust to it.

It is possible to understand how this natural adjustment works by looking for a moment at the spine. In the spine, the equivalent of plagiocephaly would be a scoliosis or crooked spine (figure 8, A & B). Again, most people have some mild asymmetry of the spine, but in some cases it is extreme. I have seen many scoliotic patients, sometimes in their 50s or 60s, who have had very little trouble with their back despite the spine condition. The abnormal curvatures

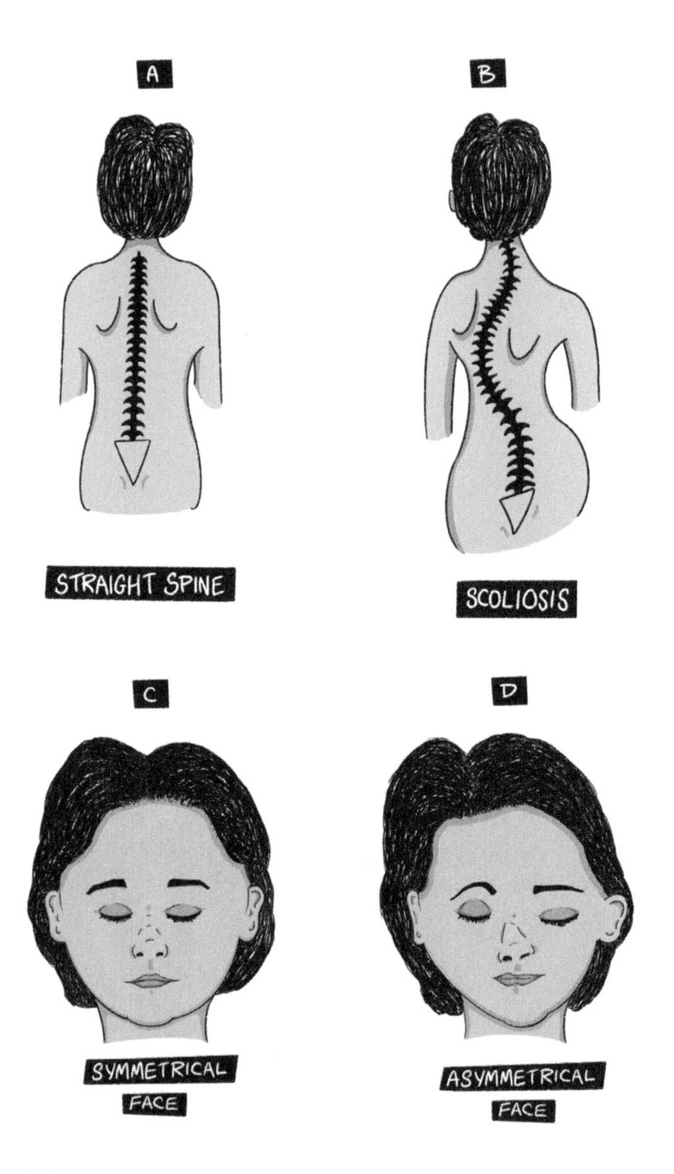

Figure 8. An example of a straight spine and a scoliotic spine (above) and a symmetrical and asymmetrical face (below). Note how the asymmetry of the scoliotic spine reflects into the shoulder and pelvic girdles (B). The asymmetry of the face (and vault) is often a reflection of a 'scoliotic' cranial base (D).

'reflect' into their shoulders and pelvic girdle and somehow the different parts of the body have found a way to work harmoniously. The body has found an effective 'compensatory mechanism' for the imbalances. A particular problem for these patients however is that if they suffer some form of subsequent injury, perhaps a car accident, it can lead to a breakdown in the existing, delicately balanced, compensation. Their back starts to hurt for the first time. It can be much harder for these patients to recover, to restore their previous balance.

The same problem experienced by scoliotic patients applies to patients with plagiocephaly (figure 8, C & D). A visible imbalance in the face or skull can be no problem whatsoever, so long as the different parts of the three-dimensional jigsaw puzzle of the skull have found a way of sitting comfortably in relationship to each other. Remember that all the different parts have grown and formed around one another since conception. However, in some cases plagiocephaly is a problem. This is especially so if the skull has previously adapted to the asymmetry and then there is some form of additional trauma to their plagiocephalic skull, such as a bang on the head from a fall or a dental or surgical procedure to the head or face.[22]

In a clinical situation, where an adult patient with plagiocephaly has come for an osteopathic consultation and is complaining of a mental health problem, how does the osteopath know if the mood disorder is connected with abnormal housing of the brain – that membrain disorder might be a contributory factor? It can't be done just by looking. The answer is by palpating the head.

PALPATION

It is possible to feel a pulse through the skin of a wrist or neck by 'palpating' the artery below. At its simplest, palpation means using a sense of touch to perceive something which can't be seen with the eyes. The word comes from the Latin *palpare*, to touch gently, and most people will recognise it from going to a GP or A&E with a suspected bone fracture, painful rib or possible appendicitis. The doctor will gently press the affected area and get an initial impression (sometimes admittedly from your cries of pain rather than through their fingers) of what feels abnormal. Typically, the next stage for medical GPs and consultants is tests by machines like X-Rays and MRIs that can 'see' through the skin in a way the human eye cannot.

For osteopaths, and manual therapists in general, palpation is far, far, more than this kind of brief exploratory pressing of the skin. Palpation is an active skill, central to the practice of osteopathy and developed by the practitioner over years of training and professional practice. Osteopaths trained in the specialist cranial field can, believe it or not, palpate not only through the skin covering the skull but through the many fine bones of the skull to the directly underlying tough membrane system, the dura. The dura is highly reactive and if there is a problem it is possible to palpate this 'reaction' – in other words, to 'see' with one's hands what is going on under the surface. Palpation through the bony cranium is one of the crucial skills that students start to learn on the challenging Osteopathy in the Cranial Field postgraduate courses.

So palpation has a diagnostic aspect (discovering what's going on), but what's really significant is that it also shows a way of treating the problem (of influencing what's going on). In the human body every system, big or small (whether a liver, a kidney, a muscle, a blood vessel, and so on), is wrapped in membrane like the dura, often called fascia. Fascia is a bag around an area, one which also connects it to other areas of the body. Importantly, fascia is a living tissue, rich in nerve receptors and highly responsive to its living environment. As such, it is possible for an appropriately trained manual practitioner to influence the fascia of any organ or area in the body via an indirect manual contact; to influence the housing of that system. The arteries, veins and the accompanying nerves that supply an organ enter via tunnel-like channels also formed by the fascia. So, in influencing the fascia, a practitioner is not only altering the housing but also influencing the vital circulatory channels feeding the area it encloses (figure 9).

THE FASCIA

Fascia literally means 'face' or 'surface'. When dissecting a body from the outside in, the first surface encountered when getting to an organ or area is the membrane which wraps round it – the fascia. Historically in a dissection this 'surface' would always be peeled away and left in a bucket under the table while only the contents it housed were examined! It is only relatively recently that it has become more apparent to medical scientists what an extremely important role the fascia plays in health and disease in various parts of the body.[23] Yet this is knowledge that osteopaths have used in treating patients for more than a century.

In this book the focus is just on the midline axis of the body's extensive fascial system – namely the dura (figure 4). This midline axis is the tadpole-shaped dural membrane or dura mater, the head of which houses the brain. Within this, the book is focusing on just one aspect of the dura, its connection with mental health. The points made above about fascia in general apply equally to the specific area of the brain and the dura that surrounds it. A manual therapist can influence the tadpole-shaped membrane system, the dura, through an indirect manual contact, influencing not only the housing of the brain but also the circulatory channels supplying the brain.

MEDICINE OR MAGIC?

At first glance it might seem inconceivable that a practitioner, however skilled in palpation of other softer parts of the body, can really feel a flexible membrane through the hard bone of the skull,

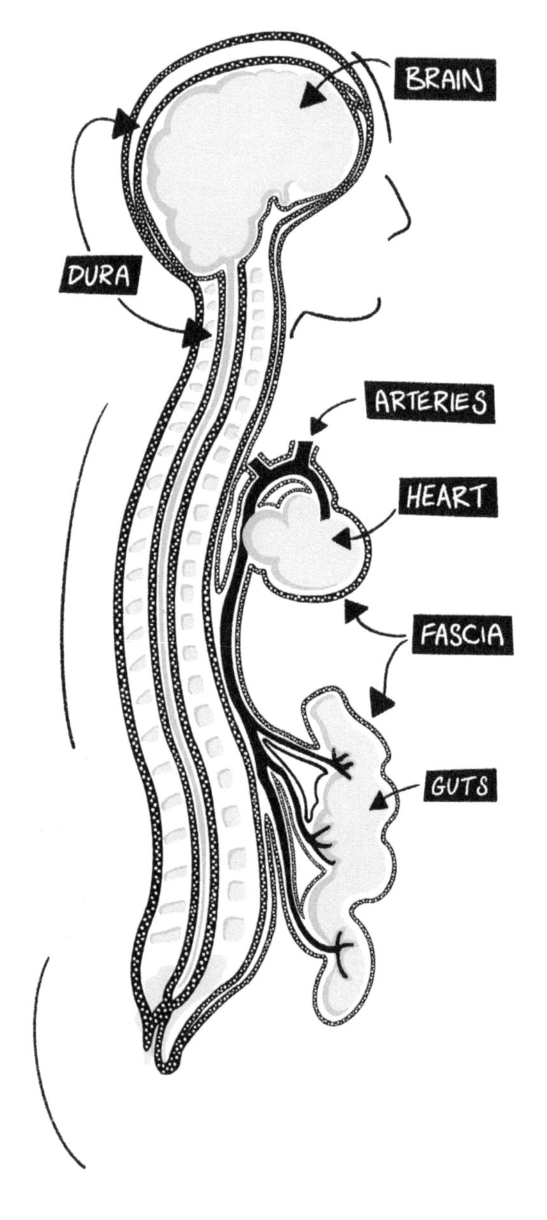

Figure 9. A continuous fascial system providing compartments for the organs, channels for the blood vessels to and from the organs, and connectivity between the organs.

let alone treat it. Surely the hard bone masks any sensation of the softer membranous material of the dura? But this is to confuse feeling with palpation.

A rather simplistic example might help. One can imagine a thin, flat, plywood board, about the size of an iPad, glued tightly to the top of a small foam cushion about the same size. The board represents the bony skull, the foam cushion the dural membrane. By gently pressing down on and then gradually releasing the board (that is, palpating it), one will feel the movement of the cushion below. In fact, it's impossible to miss it. Although the fingers are touching only the board, most of what is felt is the movement of the cushion. The springiness of the cushion, its resistance to being pressed down in the centre, the different angle and feeling of resistance sensed near the edges, the direction and strength of its rebound and so on, are all discernible by touch. In fact, with a bit of practice it is possible to get to know the properties of the foam cushion pretty well without ever seeing it or touching it directly.

Such an example can only go so far. The body is not glued together from inert materials like plywood and foam. The main reason that one can not only feel the membrane system through the bones of the skull but also influence it – treat it – is that the skull and dura are, in reality, different forms of the same 'connective tissue' system. They share a common origin and are intricately related. It is impossible to influence one part without influencing the others.

EVERYTHING CONNECTS

An anatomy book will separate a ligament from a muscle, a muscle from a bone, the skull from the dura and so on and give them all separate names.[24]

These different names in reality describe a continuous living substance that has developed from the embryonic state and is simply more condensed in some areas than others – this continuous living substance is the connective tissue system. The bone, very dense and therefore relatively hard, is the most condensed area. The blood is the least condensed and takes a fluid form. Blood, blood vessels, muscles, bone, ligaments and the fascia are all part of a continuous connective tissue system that provides nutrition, support, compartmentalisation and continuity to the different organs of the body.

These combined connective tissues all develop from the mesoderm, the middle layer of a three-layer disc present at the very earliest embryological stage during the development of the human form in the womb.

Each reader of this book was, once, about twelve days after fertilization of the egg from which they originated, a three-layered disc (figure 10). The upper layer represents the future central nervous system (CNS) and skin. The lower layer is the future digestive system (a continuous tube that starts at the mouth and finishes at the anus). The middle layer represents the future connective tissue system. The ongoing development of the upper and lower layers is completely reliant on the middle layer for stimulus in the form of information and nourishment and for the development of shape and positioning by restraint and containment.

The intimate interrelationship of these three layers never changes at any stage through development, birth and growth, right up to the end of one's life, despite increasing levels of complexity as the full human form develops over the months, years and decades. The middle layer, the connective tissue, becomes the environment of the central nervous system (CNS) and the digestive system. The health and the behaviour of the CNS and digestive system are entirely reliant on their shared environment of the connective tissue system.

DIAGNOSIS BY PALPATION

By feeling through the skull, then, the practitioner can palpate the

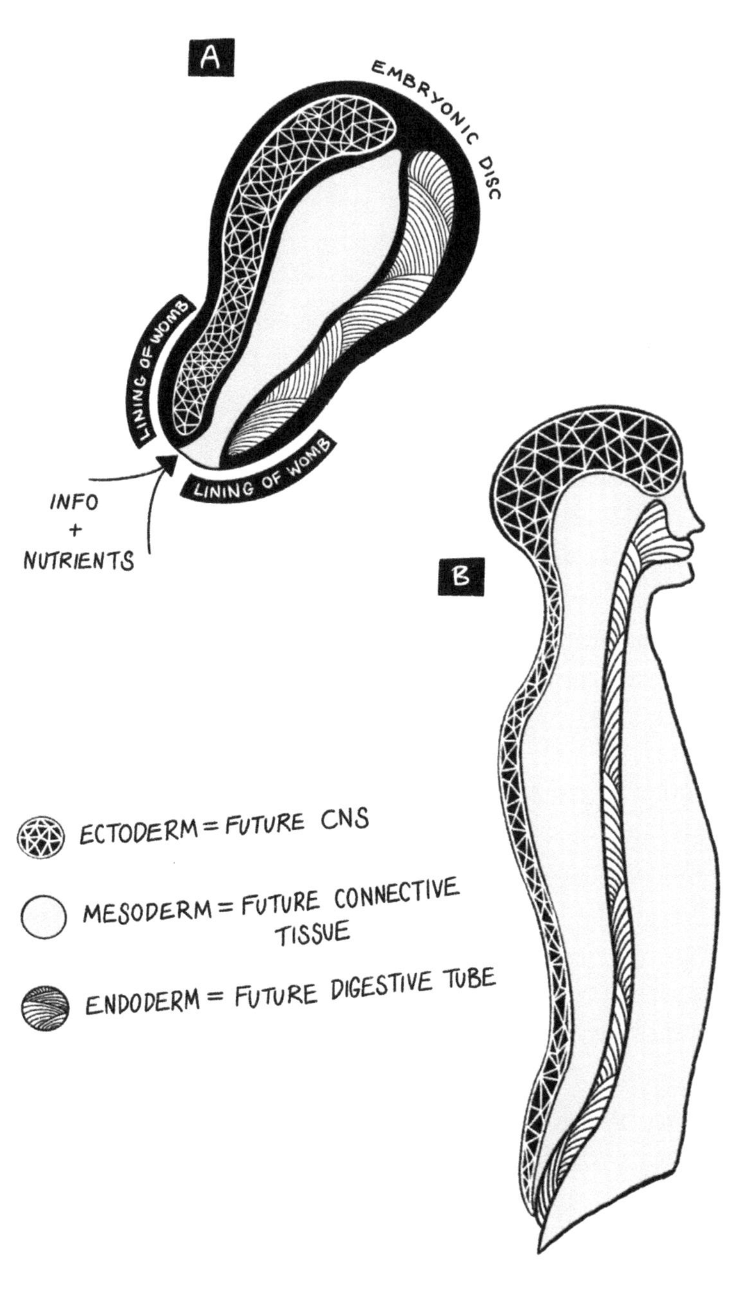

Figure 10. Trilayer embryonic disc (A) and trilayer adult (B)

dura, the tadpole-shaped membrane structure, just as with the board and foam cushion. The dura is difficult to feel when there is not a problem: when the dura is not reactive, or, to put it another way, it has no story to tell. However, when the twenty-two bones of the three-dimensional jigsaw of the skull are not sitting comfortably in relationship to one another, it will be the dura that reacts to try to set things right and this reaction, this change, can be palpated.

What is going on within the skull is similar to the way a muscle reacts to a twisted knee or a disc injury in the lower back. The reaction there is visible in the way a damaged joint is held protectively; the knee will not straighten or the patient will be unable to stand upright because of contracting muscles around the damaged area. The muscles are hard and are pulling in a certain direction. In the case of the skull, such pulls are not visible but a suitably trained practitioner can palpate a combination of reactivity, quality and change in shape of the dura. This change in shape of the dura creates 'pulls' at the points of its attachment to the skull. The practitioner can then interact with the dura and effect a treatment.

GOING BACK TO FREDDIE

I will never forget that day in my practice when I placed my hands on Freddie's head, palpating beneath the bones through to the underlying dura: absolute chaos. The behaviour of the membrane system was the most erratic I have ever felt. The housing of Freddie's brain was in extreme distress.

I have since observed many markedly asymmetrical faces in the photographs of celebrities staring out at me from magazines and television, individuals who are known to live with bipolar disorder and other psychological conditions. The housing of the brain may or may not be a contributory factor in their mental health history, but if membrain disorder is a factor, someone with the correct training and a certain way of thinking might be able to help or, in more tragic cases, might have been able to help.

FOUR

HEAD TRAUMA AND MEMBRAIN DISORDER

George's story

"I am sorry," I said, "I don't treat patients with psychosis."

George's mother was persistent. She had heard of my success in treating patients with mental health conditions and she was determined to get to the bottom of what had happened to her son. He was not responding to the prescribed medication and she had an instinctive feeling that the psychotic episode he was currently experiencing was somehow linked to earlier head trauma.

I explained again that I couldn't treat her son, but she insisted that as medical professionals themselves, she and her husband could provide the support network needed while George went through any treatment with me.

"Please, please see him."

George came for an initial consultation a week later. He was in his early twenties, a young man who appeared physically well and fit but who was alarmingly absent. His body was right there in front of me, but whoever was inside that body had been removed entirely.

His mother described his symptoms: forgetful, distant, confused, depressed, a poor sleeper, no energy, no goals, smoking, anger and disgust displayed towards women.

"Tell me about the head trauma?"

When he was six years old, George had been hanging upside down on the monkey bars in his local park. His hands slipped and he plunged down, his head taking the full impact of the fall. He had fractured his skull. Two years later George was involved in another accident when he was kicked in the forehead during a collision in a game of football. He appeared to recover well after both accidents. The year before coming for this consultation, George had endured yet another blow to his head, falling backwards onto concrete, striking the back of his head this time.

There was no history of mental health disorders in the family and George himself had been a cheerful, engaged, active child. He had never suffered with a psychological illness growing up but during the last year he had changed.

On visual examination all looked normal. There were no signs of the plagiocephaly I had seen in Freddie (chapter 3). However, on palpating George's head, all was not normal.

The dura had a story to tell.

In George, the dura displayed a sensitivity so acute that it did not allow touch. In these situations, which practitioners in this field come to recognise, there is a deep sense of discomfort – on the part of the practitioner – and an overwhelming sense of being repulsed or pushed away by a disturbed physiological activity from the particular area that needs to be explored. In George's case this was the entire head, the cranium, that had been subject to the historical traumas.

The sensitivity signified a physiological system in deep distress and a self-repair system working frantically but unsuccessfully to self-correct. The capability of a body to self-repair and the effort that the body puts into this is so often forgotten. But it is there, and it has many different genius forms: inherent self-healing and self-regulating mechanisms.

Besides the well-known immune system which fights viruses and infections, there is also a structural system which will organise itself in order to allow repair to damage. Muscles will contract around the strained ligament of a knee or a disc damage of the spine in a way that protects the damaged area, allowing it to heal. The membrane system under our skull, the dura, behaves in the same way. It will 'pull' on an area, using its points of attachment to the skull, if positional or functional relationships have been disturbed.

The behaviour of the membrane system is corrective; it will work to return things to normal. If the membrane system has been in a corrective state over a long period of time and yet failing, it will become fatigued, agitated, or sensitised. In Freddie, the young man diagnosed with schizophrenia mentioned in chapter 3, the dura was agitated in an extreme way. In George it was sensitised in an extreme way. The two different feelings in the membrane system are evident to the experienced practitioner.

Because of the extreme sensitisation of George's dura I could not put my hands directly on his head for the first couple of treatments. I started work at the tail end of the tadpole-shaped structure, its lower pole of attachment down at the pelvis. The dura is one whole structure enveloping both the brain and the spinal cord, so it is possible to influence the whole dural system from different points of contact.

Eventually, after a couple of sessions, the dura settled and I was able to rest my hands on George's head and get a sense of what was going on. His right parietal bone (covering most of the upper right side of the head) was compressed downwards relative to its neighbours while the frontal bone (covering the forehead) was pushing backwards and upwards (figure 11). Both findings were consistent with the two head traumas – a fractured skull and kicked head – that he had experienced as a child. What I was feeling through the skull were unresolved physical traumas or 'legacies' of these impacts.

When the bones are pushed together and actually meet, the sutures (junctions) can fuse over and become solid bone. The two arrows in figure 11 demonstrate the directions of the forces that George's skull were subject to and how this might cause the compression of certain sutures. (Such localised compressions are quite visible to the naked eye when looking at old skulls.)

I treated George over a period of five months. His parents brought him each time, sat in the waiting room, took him home and kept an eye on him. He recovered steadily and by the following spring he was back at university, playing football and off medication.

After my encounter with George, whilst doing the ironing and listening with half an ear to Woman's Hour, my full attention became caught by an interview. An eminent scientist was discussing the definitive statistical link between childhood head trauma caused by accidents, such as falling out of a tree, and depression and suicide in adulthood.[25,26] It was a solemn and earnest conversation about a discovery based on careful research and the amassing of evidence. It was very relevant to my own thoughts around this subject and I was delighted to hear the link between head trauma and mental health being voiced, but as the interview went on I started to feel increasingly despondent and frustrated by the very limited scope of the discussion.

There did not seem to be any questioning of why this link existed and as a consequence there was no consideration of a possible treatment to prevent such a distressing outcome. There is a similarly proven link between adult head trauma, long standing depression, behavioural issues, criminality, substance abuse and suicide, but again no explanation for the link or suggestions for treatment to prevent these effects occurring.[27,28,29,30]

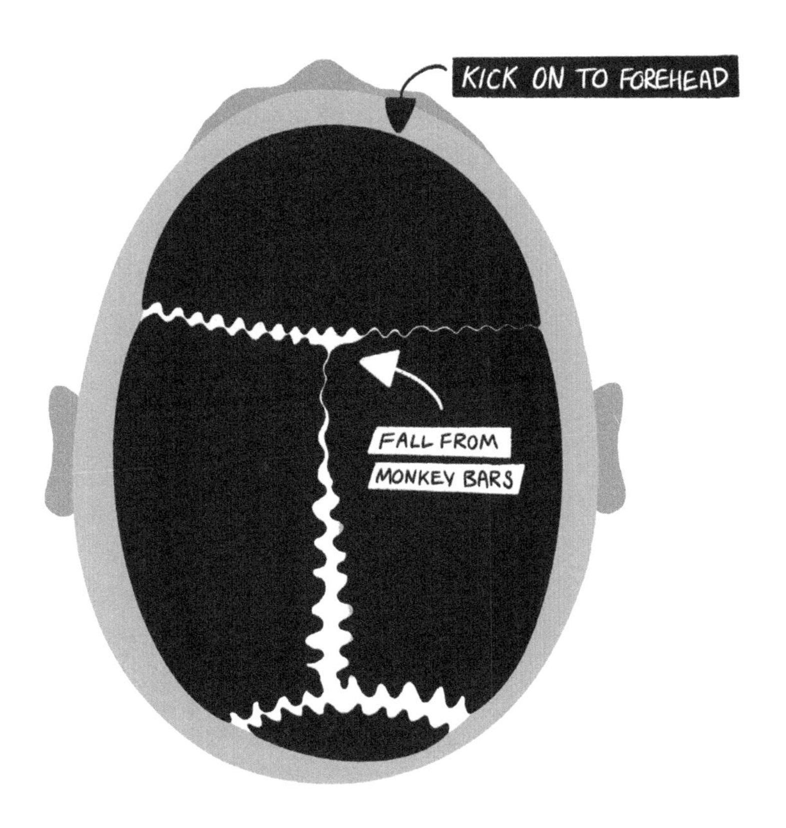

Figure 11. A view of George's skull from above.

THE MISSING LINK?

With more recent publicity surrounding the link between sports head injuries, mental health issues and dementia, the question of the physical 'missing link' that connects head injury and mental health problems across years and even decades has become even more pressing.

If the concept of membrain disorder is taken into consideration, it is possible to see that the link between accidental childhood head trauma and severe depression in later life is lasting damage inflicted not directly on the brain but on the bony skull. The damage to the skull does not have to be a fracture or some obvious bony displacement that can be picked up by X-Ray, but only a 'functional disturbance', an altered relationship between the individual bones of the skull. To use the analogy of the 3-D jigsaw, one jigsaw piece could get jammed up against and into its neighbour, creating a complex distortion (figure 12).

If the dura fails to resolve the disturbance by exerting its corrective force on the bones, the abnormal housing will persist, creating a long-term altered environment for the brain and perhaps a weakened membrane system less able to resolve any further knocks on the skull. This changed environment can have an impact on the behaviour of the brain (and hence emotions and thoughts) making individuals who have suffered a head trauma as a child more vulnerable to problems with their mental health and, as shown through scientific studies, more prone to suicide or, as in George's case, to psychosis.

All of this potentially stems from the damage only to the bony skull, not direct damage to the brain tissue itself.[31]

DELAYED ACTION

Following on from the initial short-term effects of head trauma (bruises, a mild concussion, headaches, vagueness) at a relatively young age, it is possible for the altered bony relationships of the

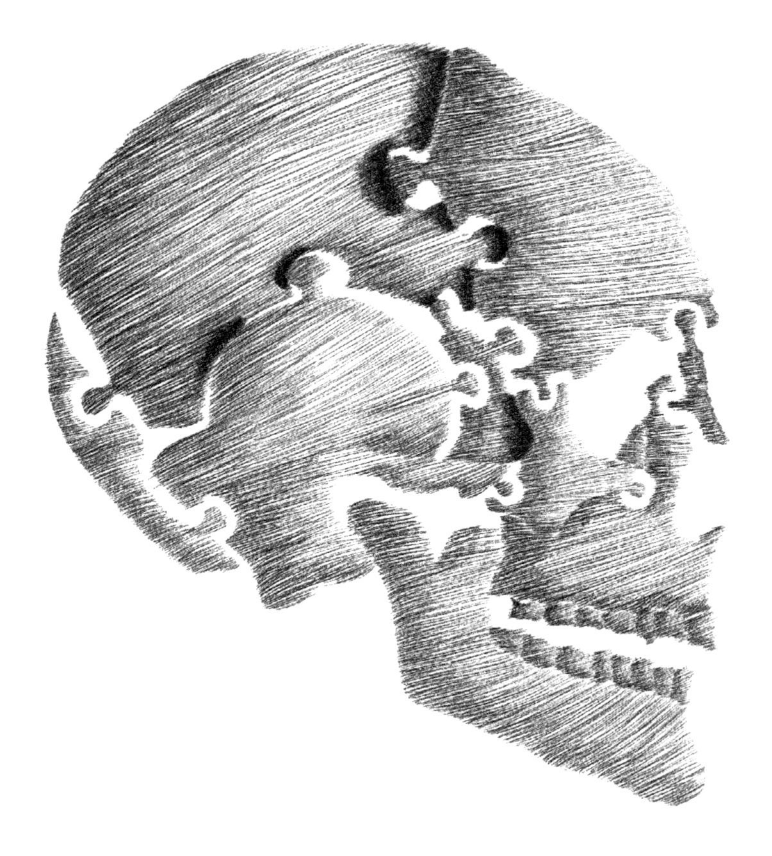

Figure 12. Jarred puzzle piece, the parietal bone

skull to remain without symptoms for years to come. The body will find a way of compensating. However, growth into adulthood, orthodontic work (to be discussed in chapter 7) or further physical injury to the head can all, individually or cumulatively, impose an extra strain on the functional disturbance which has remained since childhood and this can cause a serious problem in later years.

Children will always bang their heads. Even with helmets the head is still traumatised. These children should be examined for membrain disorder following a head trauma. If findings are positive, they should be treated in a preventive way even if they are not displaying any signs of illness subsequent to the impact on the head. For any budding young sportsmen and women developing their skills in martial arts, boxing, football, rugby, bobsleighing, skiing or any other contact sports, intermittent examination and where necessary treatment could prevent later problems.

NEW UNDERSTANDINGS OF THE BRAIN

In the early 1990s, new brain imaging techniques were revolutionising our understanding of how the brain functions. Different imaging techniques using advanced physics and computer technology allowed scientists for the first time to visualise how different parts of the brain are activated when, for example, performing certain tasks or remembering events from the past. Neuroimaging made it possible to visualise the brain as it processed memories, sensations and emotions and it became possible to map circuits and link areas of the brain according to their function.[32,33]

Knowing the location of areas of the brain associated with different emotions and behaviours means that we can identify their housing. Once it is known which cranial bones surround which areas, it is possible to visualise how the emotions associated with those areas might be influenced by membrain disorder – abnormal housing of that area of the brain in the form of a distortion of the space, decreased space, congestion, or most likely a combination of the above.[34]

Revisiting George's traumatised skull and Freddie's asymmetrical skull in light of the sick building analogy (chapter 2), one could ask: was it that the whole building was poorly designed, affecting all occupants? Or was it just one room affecting just part of the workforce, in which case, which department, which specific area of the brain, is being disturbed?

In George's case, he had fallen down from a monkey bar and fractured his skull and later had been kicked in the forehead. The forehead is the frontal bone and behind this lies the frontal lobes of the brain (figure 13). That's the first 'room'. The region of the frontal lobes of the brain is associated with consciousness, identity (a sense of 'I') and self-will. It enables focus, an ability to pay attention and to make decisions. The symptoms of schizophrenia, depression, and attention deficit disorder can be traced to overactivity or underactivity in the region of the frontal lobes.[35, 36, 37]

Beneath the right parietal bone lies the right parietal lobe of the brain (figure 14). That's a second room. The right parietal lobe is the only part of the brain that holds a 'whole' body image that it can integrate with the surrounding world, allowing a sense of connectedness.[38] Damage to this area can lead to introversion, a person who is disconnected and cut off.

Suppose membrain disorder rather than direct damage to an area of the brain itself has a similar effect? This would explain George's delayed mental suffering and offer a straightforward physical explanation for his condition. George was experiencing psychotic symptoms as a consequence of abnormal housing of the brain caused by two head injuries to the cranial vault when he was a child. The unresolved legacies of these traumas in the brain housing had weakened the dura and left him vulnerable to any further disruption and they were activated following a third head trauma as an adult.

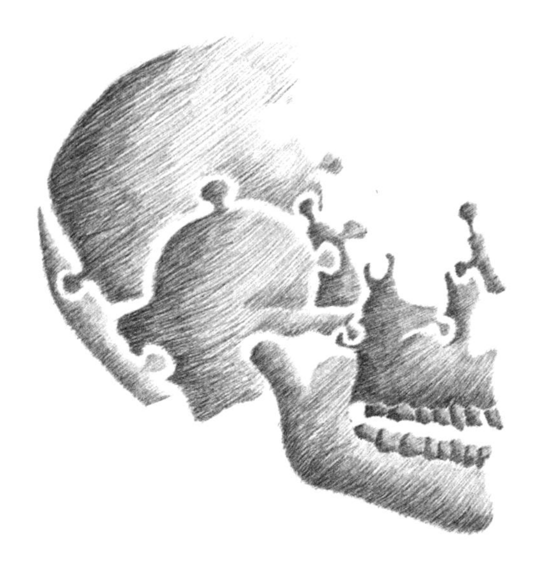

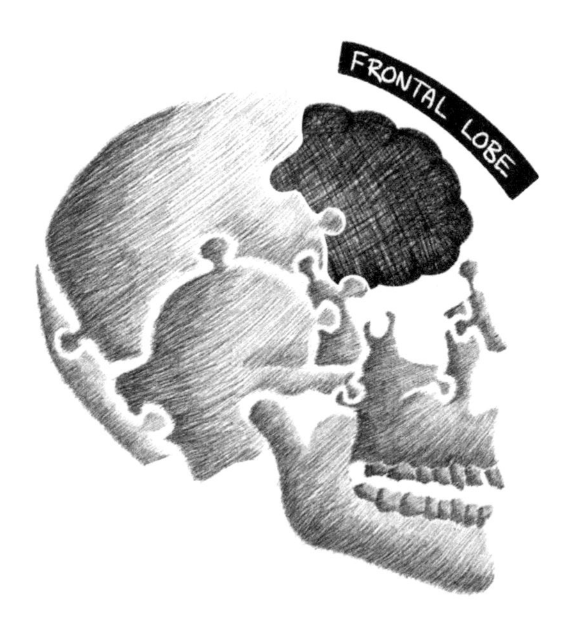

Figure 13. Skull with frontal bone removed (above), housing frontal lobe of the brain (below).

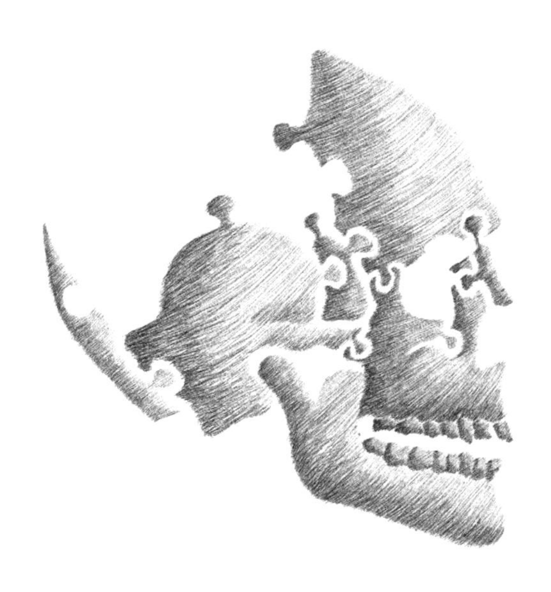

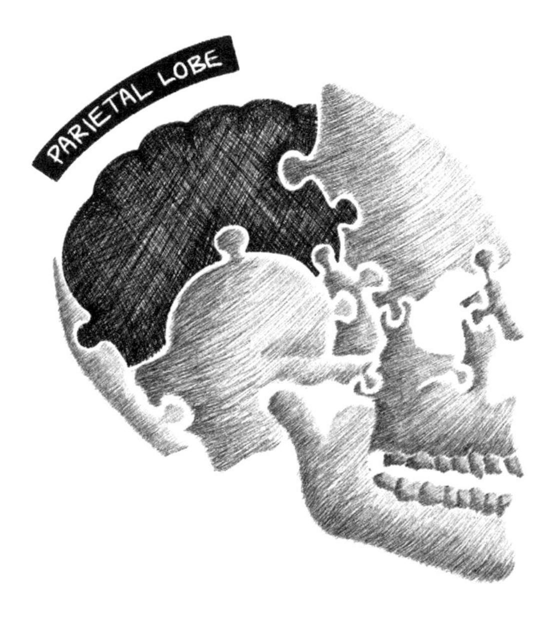

Figure 14. Skull with parietal bone removed (above) housing parietal lobe of brain (below).

It is a case of one layer of damage, then another layer of damage, and then the third layer of damage to the brain's housing is too much for the body, in the form of the dura, to cope with – it is the straw that breaks the camel's back. Manual therapists call this a 'breakdown in compensation', since in the first two cases the body successfully compensated for (adapted to) the skull injuries. The third time round, the overworked dura couldn't cope.

However, diagnosing the problem is only part of the story. There is also a route towards getting George better, if the dura can be helped to recover its strength, release the historical strain of past traumas on his skull and as far as possible restore normal housing.

But how can one treat a skull?

FIVE

HOW TO TREAT A SKULL

Amy

We met Amy briefly in the Introduction to this book. Amy's parents were at the point of taking the psychiatrist's advice to medicate their daughter in an attempt to stop something awful happening. Amy, thirteen years old at the time, was developing intensely bad feelings towards classmates and becoming incapable of controlling herself. She demonstrated this in violence towards her fellow pupils. There was no obvious trigger for her aggression nor a particular target at which it was directed and she had been excluded from school as a consequence of her behaviour. Her parents were confounded and at their wits' end.

Amy had other strange characteristics. When she knew she had behaved badly she would revert to the behaviour of a small child, hiding her face in the back of a sofa and rocking softly, vulnerable and full of shame.

Amy's parents brought her to see me at the suggestion of another patient. Amy was in the early stages of puberty. She seemed a gentle, mild mannered and slightly apprehensive girl. Her mother talked openly in front of her about how worried they all were and how nothing seemed to be preventing the situation from getting worse and worse.

I listened to them both and heard nothing that seemed significant in terms of the membrain health concept. There was no history of birth trauma, childhood head trauma or any orthodontic work. Observing Amy across the desk, I saw no signs of plagiocephaly. It was not looking as if an osteopathic approach would be of much help in this situation.

It was not until I examined Amy's skull with my hands that I became aware of the dura pulling strongly and condensing towards a point above the inside of her right eyebrow. I looked more closely at this area and there was a small faint scar. It was only when I pointed it out that the mother suddenly remembered; there had been a fall, when Amy was about two years old, onto the sharp corner of a radiator. There had been a lot of blood, Amy had been taken to hospital, been given the all clear and then the accident had been forgotten.

BASIC INSTINCTS AND THE 'CONSCIOUS' BRAIN

The area located just behind Amy's scar is part of the frontal lobe of the brain and is involved in the suppression of basic instincts.[39] These basic instincts themselves, our survival instincts, are located deep in the skull in what is called our unconscious brain. These instincts include appetite, sexual urges and aggression, amongst others. 'Unconscious' simply means that a person is unaware of the activity going on in this 'primitive' part of the brain. It has a similar design to that found in reptiles, a group of animals that has existed for over 300 million years, which is why this part of the brain is referred to as 'reptilian'.

When these 'primitive' instincts come to the surface, it is part of the brain that emerged way further along the evolutionary path, the *cerebral hemispheres*, that allows us to take control of these urges and in many cases suppress them. In a frightening situation, when the impulse is to run away as fast as possible, it is possible to control this urge and consciously stand firm and face the ordeal. In an annoying situation, when the impulse is perhaps to hit someone in anger, it is possible to grit one's teeth, clench one's fists, count to ten, push back the impulse and avoid a physical confrontation. A primitive desire to accost some highly attractive person on a daily commute is untimely and inappropriate and, assuming that alcohol has not been drunk and that part of the brain which allows some conscious control is fully functioning, such actions can be avoided.

This function of suppression or management of the instinctual urges raging in the primitive or unconscious brain can be attributed, predominantly, to the frontal lobes in an area known as the *pre-frontal cortex*. This area helps a person avoid taking risks and doing stupid things but it develops slowly from birth and is not fully formed until the late twenties – a fact often only realised on looking back!

When the frontal lobes are not working properly the instinctual urges can go unchecked. In the case of anger and sexual urges the outcome can be antisocial, sometimes criminal behaviour.

There is the very famous case of Phineas Gage, a nineteenth-century railwayman who was injured as a result of a mistimed explosion. A steel rod passed upwards through his left cheek and eye and out through his forehead (figure 15). It took out a large part of his frontal lobe. He survived but changed from a capable industrious man into a social misfit. The doctor who treated him described him as follows: "... a child in his intellectual capacity and manifestations yet with the animal passions of a strong man". He had a complete inability to direct or control himself. Women were advised to stay well clear of him.[40]

Phineas Gage is an extreme example of severe damage to the forebrain.

In Amy's case it seems that the abnormal housing of the right

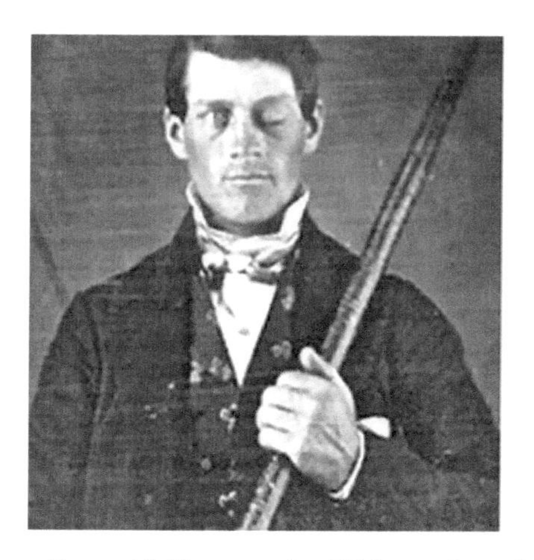

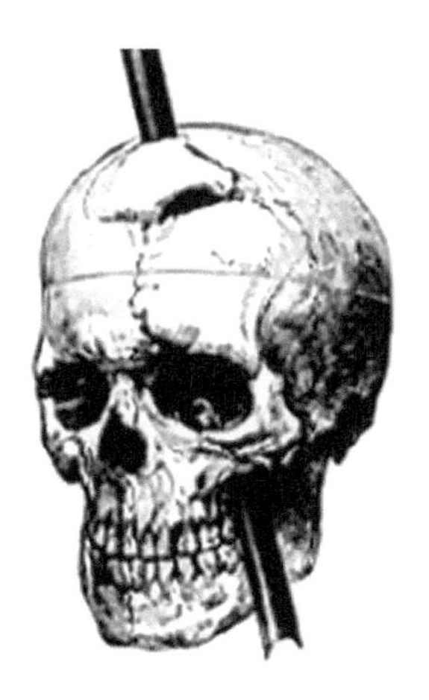

Figure 15. Photograph of Phineas Gage (left) and drawing representing the injury to his skull (right)

frontal lobe was having an impact on its behaviour; the frontal lobe was not managing to do its job properly. The symptoms were a far milder version of Phineas Gage's. I could see a scar, I could palpate a distortion in the underlying membrane system and I knew that this part of the skull had suffered an injury, albeit a long time ago.

TIME DOES NOT HEAL EVERYTHING

"A long time ago" is relevant. The fact that this injury had happened eleven years before and the trauma to the living tissue had clearly never resolved itself meant that Amy's whole system had, since her accident, grown and developed around that trauma. Conventional thinking is that the older a trauma, the less significant it is. In fact the reverse is often true; the older an unresolved trauma, the more significant it can be and the more established it is. Patients often tell me of horrendous accidents but then dismiss them as irrelevant because they happened "years ago" and "nothing was broken". Quite the reverse is often true – these can be highly significant events that the body has yet to resolve.

Perhaps surprisingly, minor injuries to the skull can sometimes be more damaging than major traumas. If an accident results in a fracture or dislocation somewhere in the body, the force of the accident is to large extent dissipated and it is often not so easy to pick up the legacy of the impact through palpation. If, however, the body has been subjected to a trauma but nothing has been broken or dislocated, the force of the trauma will not have been dissipated and is instead absorbed into the soft tissue structures. Force always has to go somewhere; it does not just disappear. This is why repeated minor knocks can have such serious consequences down the line.

Having found a problem in the skull, the next question is how to treat it? The answer is by manual therapy.

TREATMENT BY A MANUAL THERAPIST TRAINED IN THE CRANIAL FIELD

The term 'manual therapist' covers a very broad range of professions but in the literal sense it means a therapist who treats with their hands. In the context of this book 'manual therapist' refers to osteopaths, chiropractors and physiotherapists, all of whom have an extensive training comprising a four- to five-year full-time course to the level of a Bachelor (BSc) or Master of Science (MSc) degree from a validated educational institution. Students studying for each of these three professions receive a comprehensive medical training as a foundation on which to build their practical and theoretical expertise in the bio-mechanical aspects of the human body – one might say they are training to be medical body engineers.

A specialist postgraduate programme for practitioners in the field of membrain disorder is currently being developed with different pathways reflecting the aptitude and experience of students. To understand the concept of membrain health and to treat membrain disorder a practitioner has to understand the osteopathic philosophy of health, which is different from an orthodox view. The osteopathic philosophy of health relies far more heavily on the body's inherent ability to heal itself and sees the practitioner as there just to give a (highly skilled) helping hand or to remove an obstacle that is hindering the body's self-healing ability. "*Pro natura et veritate*" ("According to Nature and Truth") was the motto of the British School of Osteopathy.[41]

A manual therapist able to treat membrain disorder needs to understand the osteopathic philosophy of health, to embrace it and to be trained and experienced in the cranial field. He or she also requires a comprehensive knowledge of the anatomy of the brain and of cognitive neuroscience. Patients with mental health problems possibly involving membrain disorder will want to check that their practitioner has been trained to a sufficient level in this speciality.

There are certain things that all manual therapists have in common. One is a thorough knowledge of anatomy. Anatomy is a branch of natural science which deals with the structural organization of living things. Human anatomy can range from the 'gross anatomy' of the whole form of a particular section of the body, including all its constituent parts (e.g. the arm, the legs, the eyes), to the 'systemic anatomy' of specific aspects of the body in the form of an organ as part of a system (heart and blood vessels, kidneys and bladder, all the skeletal muscles, and so on). Finally, there is microscopic anatomy (blood cells, nerve cells, muscle tissue, etc.). Manual therapists tend to share an extremely detailed knowledge of the musculoskeletal system, the system of muscles, skeleton, ligaments and fascia that supports and transports us – knowledge reinforced on a daily basis by their practical work.

Another thing manual therapists have in common is that they use their hands and work via the musculoskeletal system to make a change.

There are broadly two hands-on approaches – 'direct' and

'indirect' – that a manual therapist can use to effect a 'mechanical' change in a patient's body.

The most widely used category is the 'direct' approach.

DIRECT APPROACH

In the direct approach, a physical barrier in the tissue or area to be treated is 'confronted'. For example, a stiff joint is moved by articulating it (stretching it open) or, if the joint is locked, it is released with what is called a high velocity thrust technique (commonly described as a 'click'), which more or less springs the clenched-up elements apart. Another example would be stretching a shortened muscle, either lengthways or pushing across the shortened muscle fibres. Force coming from the therapist is directed to push through the restrictive barrier of the mechanical tissue in the patient. Energy is being introduced into the system from outside (figure 16). This can be an effective form of treatment for many problems.

INDIRECT APPROACH

The alternative to the above is to work with the 'indirect' approach, a manual approach that involves no force or sudden movements. In the indirect approach the practitioner works 'with' the tissues rather than 'confronting' them. If a muscle is contracting and therefore shortened, the practitioner of the indirect approach will aim, paradoxically, to bring the two ends of the muscle even nearer towards one another, in the same direction that the shortening is occurring. The technical term is to 'meet the pull'. The muscle is pulling or tensing in a certain direction in an effort to self-correct and by helping it along the muscle has less to do itself. This is taking energy out of the system.

The practitioner will then have to wait until the tissues of the patient respond. During this time nerve signals from the muscle to the brain will be changing, calming down, and the brain will correspondingly alter its message back out to the muscle. The effect is what is called a 'reflex change'. The nervous pathway of feedback loops between muscle and brain will change and, if it works, the muscle will relax and therefore lengthen again (figure 16).

The body is inherently intelligent in that it knows how to self-correct. This process of self-correction is visible to the naked eye; a cut will heal, a sprained joint will swell and then slowly recover, and a fracture will bind – over time. But at times the body needs a helping hand when the self-correction is incomplete. This is the thinking behind an 'indirect' approach.

A practitioner who works using indirect techniques relies on the intelligence and effectiveness of the patient's self-correcting mechanisms. Indirect techniques first use palpation to feel and understand what the body is trying to do to correct itself. The practitioner will then support, encourage and amplify whatever the body is seeking to do, in whatever direction it is occurring. To do this successfully, one has to spend some of the time just 'listening' to the body through the hands to understand what the body is trying to do. Some of the hand movements used in the indirect approach are hardly noticeable to an observer. For example, if the technique involves a very slight pressure or a very subtle change in the angle of support, or when the practitioner is in 'listening' mode, it can look as though nothing is happening.

To an observer, watching a manual therapist work this way on a patient is, well, like watching paint dry! It is not showy. It might look to some people like some sort of 'spiritual healing' event. But it is not. Working this way is a practical, physical skill that is acquired over many years of training and experience.

PALPATION – LISTENING, LEARNING, WAITING

The practitioner has to learn to palpate or feel at a deep level. This can be compared to the art of listening to a Mozart concerto where one person hears the music in the whole sense while another person

DIRECT TECHINIQUE

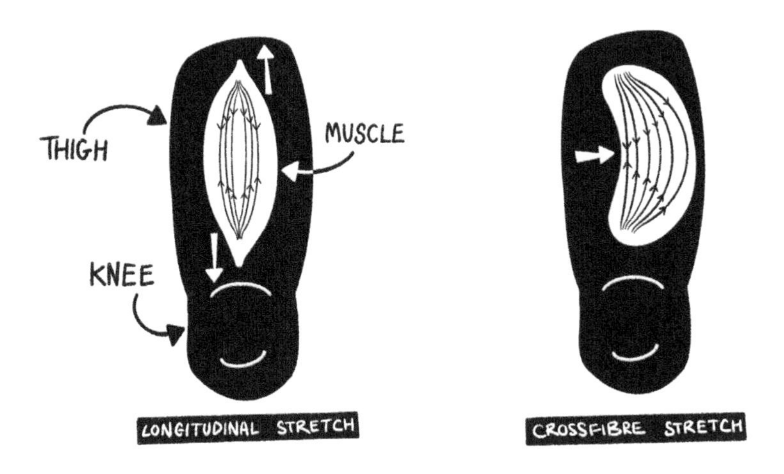

INDIRECT TECHINIQUE

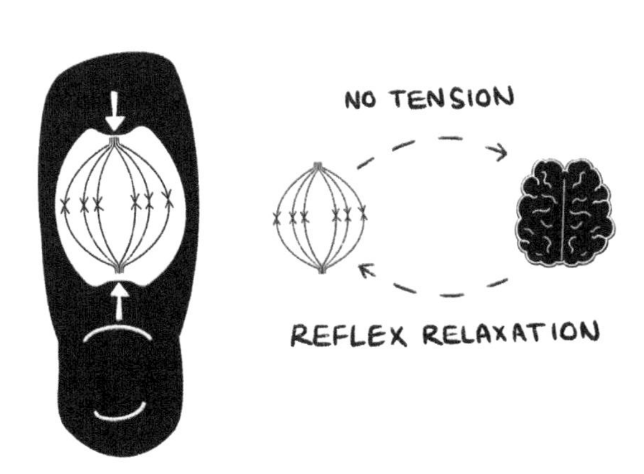

Figure 16. Illustration of direct and indirect techniques applied to the muscle of the thigh.

listens just to the violin or the wind section. Someone else may pay attention to the bass notes; others pay attention to the tempo and the range of volumes. They will hear different things, depending on what they are listening to. The subtleties of palpating can be compared to the subtleties of listening. All the different aspects one can palpate reflect the many different aspects of a complex system – and the human body is an extremely complex system.

A further skill required for the indirect technique is that of maintaining confidence that the patient's body knows best in order to be led (sometimes blindly) by 'instruction' from the patient's body. The practitioner is not the real expert here, the patient's body is. The practitioner is learning from the patient's body. A western upbringing typically does not help in appreciating the validity of this approach. Western attitudes to life, cultivated through the education system and then on into one's career, tend to value status, qualifications, decisive action, control and a 'we know best' mentality; a rather arrogant culture, looked at that way.

Learning can be seen as an attitude, one of remaining open to opportunity, continually improving one's understanding through an entire lifetime. Learning is not just a body of knowledge; it involves understanding when and how to use that knowledge appropriately. The indirect approach relies on the practitioner's ability – and willingness – to learn in that moment from a patient's body what that specific body is trying to do to correct itself – and then to help that process along. Understanding continues to develop through an entire treatment, and the next treatment, and the next. The practitioner is constantly learning from and being led by his or her patient.

A final skill and perhaps the hardest for the practitioner to master is learning to wait until those reflex changes occur (it can be seconds, or it can be minutes) and then to wait again and see what happens next. Waiting requires patience; waiting some more can really test patience.

BALANCED MEMBRANOUS TENSION

When all the bones of the three-dimensional jigsaw puzzle of the skull are sitting comfortably in relationship to one another, the dura does not become distorted. It has no need to autocorrect. If, on the other hand, there is a mismatch and discomfort somewhere among the bones, the membrane system will change its shape, creating pulls in certain directions in order to auto-correct. This is where treatment starts.

The tadpole-shaped dura condenses (it becomes thicker and heavier) where it is attached top and bottom to the bony skeleton. At the top, around the brain, the dura is attached at certain points to the inside of the skull. Down at the tail end of the tadpole it is secured to the back of the pelvis. These anchor points are known technically as 'poles of attachment' (figure 17).

It is possible, using various handholds that gently cradle the head, face and pelvis, to support the dura in its direction of pull via these poles of attachment. With skill and patience, it is possible to 'meet' the pull as described above and then wait; wait for the reflex changes that an 'indirect' technique aims to initiate through the gentle extra help that the practitioner has provided.

This procedure is known as the Balanced Membranous Tension (BMT) method. Osteopaths trained in the cranial field are adept in this method. By releasing the pull on the membrane system the biodynamics – the living physical forces – of the impacted skull will change. There may be no change of shape or structure, but things will change functionally, which is to say the various elements will come back into balance.*

* Patency of the sutures (i.e. space between the bones, as between the pieces of a jigsaw) can exist between the individual bones of the skull throughout life. From examining many skulls over the years it is apparent that when a suture is fused along a part of its length there is often a flattening of the bone, presumably from an early trauma when the bones were still quite soft. Where the joint lines are patent (open) some flexibility between the individual bones is maintained. It is not a macro-motion, nor even a micro-motion, but a small sense of 'give' between the individual bones, evidently vital for health nonetheless.

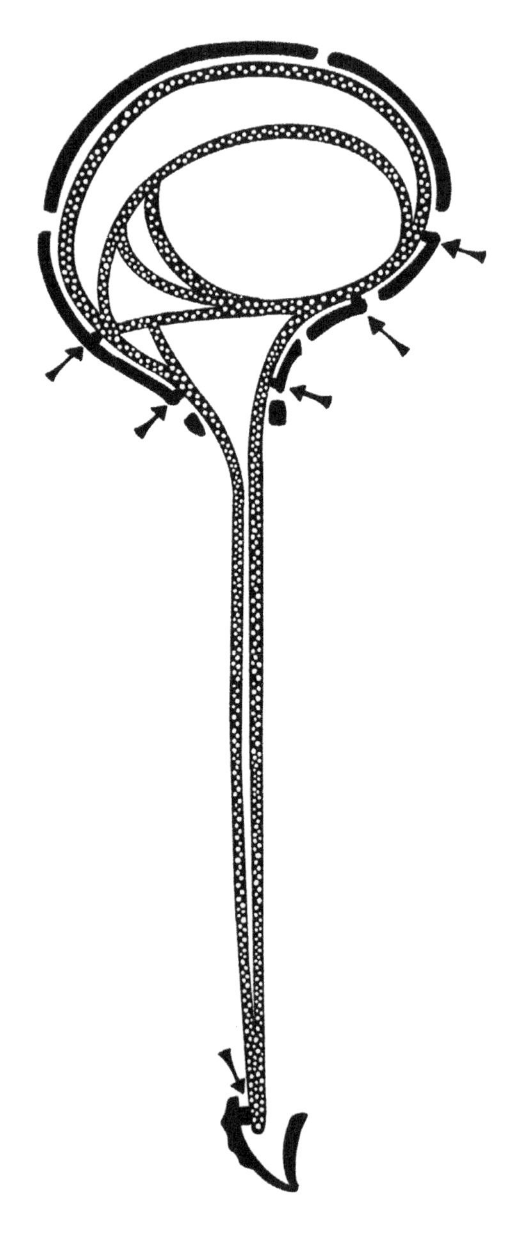

Figure 17. The points of attachment of the dura onto the bones are highlighted by the arrows. These are referred to as the 'poles of attachment' where the dura exerts its greatest influence.

A slight intervention of this kind often triggers a cascade reaction – a series of corrections. Once the therapist helps the body to get past one correction, many other corrections will often follow in sequence. The practitioner has initiated a therapeutic response; a succession of corrective actions by the body itself which will eventually restore things to their normal comfortable state.

The effect of a successful BMT treatment may on some occasions be small, limited to the immediate area being treated. Alternatively, the effect of a successful BMT session can be huge and far reaching, affecting the entire body. The therapist is working with the dura, the bag that the brain sits in and the dura is physically connected not only to the head but also to the pelvis. Effecting a change to the dura can therefore affect the behaviour of the entire central nervous system (CNS), changing the mechanics of the head and pelvis as well as the spine which connects them. The tadpole-shaped dura also represents the midline axis of the entire fascial system that houses, connects, supports and nourishes the body's organs (see figure 9). These far-reaching consequences can take hours, days, weeks or even in some cases months to fall into place after the patient has been treated.

Back to Amy

I was able to treat Amy just once for her uncontrollable aggressive behaviour before she went with her parents overseas. She was flown back over from the Middle East three months later specifically for a second treatment as the initial treatment had had such a big impact on her behaviour. On her follow-up examination, the abnormal pulls on the membrane system around the frontal cortex had resolved. The scar was still visible, but the functionality of the dura and frontal lobe under the scar area had changed. Amy was no longer suffering from membrain disorder and her mental health symptoms, the hostile feelings and aggressive behaviour towards her classmates, had faded.

The housing of Amy's brain had changed. How exactly the change in the dura went on to influence the behaviour of the brain itself and then Amy's feelings and actions was something way beyond the influence of my hands. In the end it was the body itself, with a little indirect help from the practitioner, that was able to reverse a behavioural disorder among the eighty-six billion neurons in the brain and bring things back towards normal.

SIX

THE UNKNOWN IMPACT OF DENTISTRY

Dido

Dido was 14 when she arrived at my practice. A budding young ballerina who was suffering with spinal pain that moved up and down her body, she had also developed OCD (obsessive compulsive disorder) over the last year. She could barely leave the house, overcome by the need to check the taps for dripping and see that all the windows were securely locked. Her condition was so severe that she was undergoing psychiatric treatment. She was physically fit and pretty with perfect teeth. Her teeth braces had come off six months previously after a two-year orthodontic correction programme straightening her previously crooked teeth.

It is rare for anyone to make the connection between structural work on the teeth and the onset of mental health problems. Yet structural work on the teeth can have a physical effect on the whole of the skull, whether it be a tooth extraction, a root canal procedure, an implant or – as a slower and sustained form of trauma – the application of braces to straighten one's teeth.

The upper row of teeth sits in the 'middle face' (*maxilla*) while the lower row of teeth sits in the 'lower face' or jawbone (*mandible*). Any physical change to the middle or lower face has the potential to cause membrain disorder – even temporarily. By considering the intricate relationship of the three parts of the skull – the cranial vault, the cranial base and the face – it is possible to understand that any structural work that changes the physical dynamics of the face may have an indirect impact on those parts of the skull that physically house the brain.

THE INTRICATE RELATIONSHIP OF THE FACE AND THE 'TEMPORAL BONES'

The jawbone sits suspended in a hammock-like arrangement of soft tissues (muscles, ligaments, etc.) that originate from the skull's cranial base and vault (figure 18). The jawbone is also connected via joints on either side with the left and right temporal bones (described below) – these are the temporo-mandibular joints (TMJs). All of the elements involved – soft tissue, joints, and bony structures – have grown together from the very start of life and their individual forms are compatible, meaning that as they have grown they have adapted to any minor irregularities to function well together as a unit.

THE TEMPORAL BONES

The temporal bones have a nickname in the osteopathic profession which is 'the troublemakers'. As a pair they form part of both the cranial vault and the cranial base and connect directly with the bones of the middle and lower face. Each temporal bone (figure 19) has seven neighbouring bones. It is collectively their job to reconcile the three parts of the cranium – to keep it working well. The intricacies in the design details of the joint lines between a temporal bone and the seven other adjoining bones are a complex beauty to behold and reflect the extraordinary and delicate relationships this bone has with its neighbours.

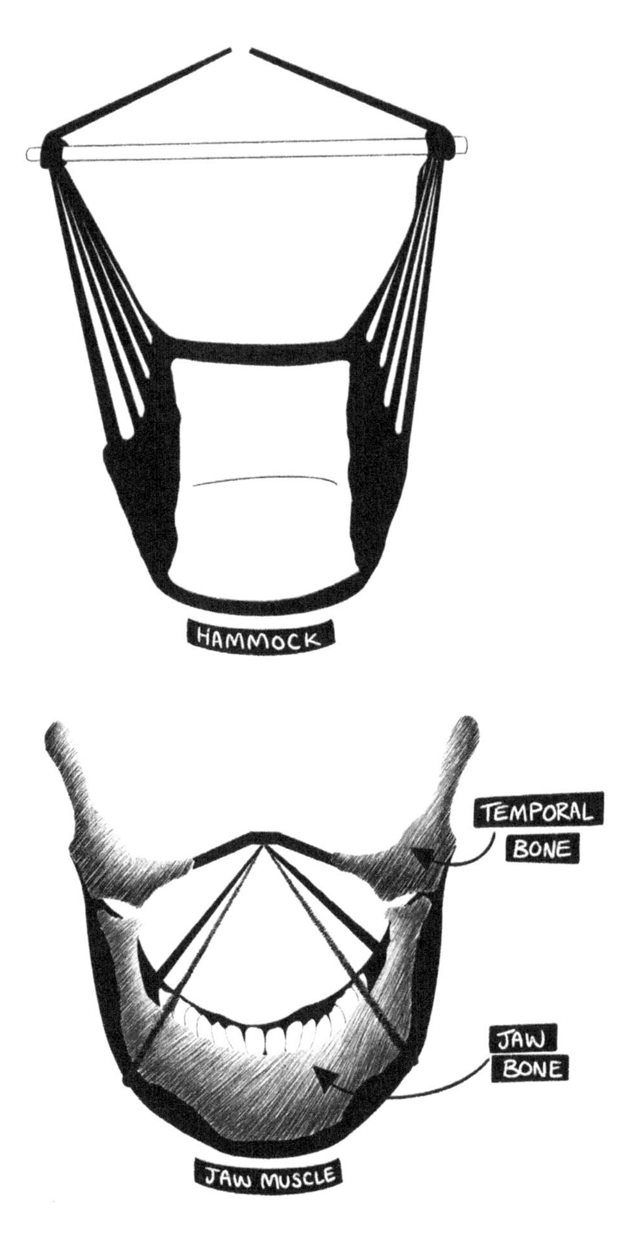

Figure 18. (Above) A hammock system. (Below) A jawbone as it sits in the hammock system of muscles and ligaments suspended from the cranial base and both sides of the cranial vault.

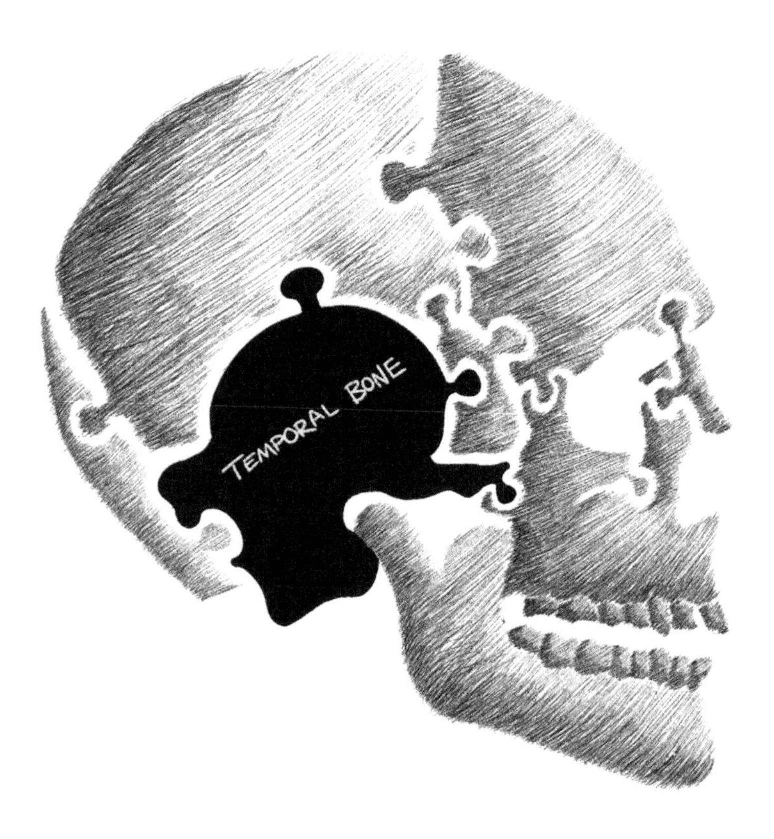

Figure 19. Right temporal bone in situ.

Any structural work to the lower face, including the lower array of teeth, whether by orthodontic work, a tooth extraction or jaw surgery, can have an impact on one or both of the temporal bones. Any structural work to the middle face (the upper teeth area), whether by orthodontic work, a tooth extraction or palate (roof of the mouth) surgery, may have an impact on one or both of the temporal bones and the cranial base.

The dura will react accordingly, in an attempt to reconcile the changes and find a new order in the working relationship of the twenty-two-piece jigsaw puzzle. In cases where the dura is unable to find a way to reconcile the changes, membrain disorder may be an outcome.

ORTHODONTIC WORK

A large proportion of readers may have had orthodontic work as a child, or they may have sought treatment as an adult, or they may well have seen their own children through orthodontic care.

Orthodontist literally means 'one who puts teeth right'. The aim of an orthodontist is to correct any abnormal occlusion (the way the upper and lower teeth meet to bite) and to reposition any teeth that are misaligned relative to their neighbours. A successful course of treatment would aim to create a 'perfect' occlusion and a 'perfect' set of teeth. In many cases a patient going through orthodontic treatment will have a misalignment of the bite, either already causing or having the potential to cause disfigurement, pain or problems with chewing. The other reason for orthodontic work is for cosmetic reasons: to achieve the 'ideal' smile.

Orthodontic work involves a number of different methods, as follows:

- **Teeth extractions**

  If the upper or lower jaw is too small to accommodate the permanent (adult) teeth, this leads to overcrowding of the mouth. The orthodontist will extract some teeth to give more space for the remainder.

- **Traditional wired braces**
  A wired brace is used to move the teeth directly by exerting pressure on the teeth, either tooth by tooth or as a unit.

- **Clear aligners**
  A common approach is to offer a series of braces of clear hardened plastic that are worn over the teeth and which gradually move the teeth into the perfect arch. These braces are more commonly used in older children and adults. Many adults nowadays are opting for what is called 'cosmetic dentistry' which includes teeth whitening, crowns and veneers but has increasingly moved into the realm of orthodontics and the frequent use of clear aligners.

- **Retainers**
  Whatever approach is used to provide the perfect dental arch, and at whatever age this is done, once the teeth are in position and the occlusion is as perfect as the dentist can make it, the patient is commonly asked to wear retainers. These can take the form of a brace worn at night or alternatively a permanent wire is fixed onto the back of the teeth where it is invisible, sometimes both top and bottom. This is to stop the teeth from moving back (through the self-correcting efforts of the body) to the position whence they came.

- **Palatal expanders**
  In expansion work, an orthodontist works over a period of time on the bony development of the upper or lower jaws, gradually helping the palate and/or the jaw to broaden

laterally and forwards. The idea is to help the body achieve the maximum genetic potential of possible growth. This development is encouraged by a contraption that looks like a traditional brace worn in the mouth, but it exerts pressure not on the teeth but on the bones that are the foundations of the teeth, pushing from inside outwards. Expansion work was first introduced by a group of dentists in the UK known as 'functional orthodontists'.* This group met initially with huge opposition from conventional orthodontists but their techniques have been slowly recognised and adopted over the last two decades and expansion work is now widely available.

Some orthodontists recognise the need to start expansion work from a very early age (in some cases as early as age 5 but more commonly around age 7). There is still significant plasticity in the bones at this early stage of life. The expansion work is directed at the bones, not at the individual teeth and its aim is nearly always to encourage the growth of the bones forwards and laterally, avoiding any form of compression or restriction to the face. The work is done slowly and gradually. The ability of the rest of the skull to adapt to these changes is far greater than in forced structural changes imposed later in life, perhaps in adolescence or – as is increasingly common – in adults.

Another and wonderful aspect of expansion work is that it broadens and lowers the palate. The palate forms the roof of the mouth which is one and the same as the floor of the nasal cavity located behind the nose. The nasal cavity expands in volume through the expansion procedure. The

* Functional orthodontists work by using mouth appliances to expand the bones of the middle and lower face to make more room to accommodate the teeth, to improve the way the teeth fit together (the occlusion) and to open up the airway system.

outcome is a child who will grow into an adult who can breathe nasally, and so breathe correctly. That is about the greatest gift of health that can be given to any child: a gift that will last them through adulthood and into old age – a good lifelong supply of oxygen! There are many books being published at the moment promoting the advantages of good breathing to get oxygen to the brain to help mental health and prevent degenerative brain and other diseases developing.[42] Oxygen has to come into the body and the best way is via an expansive nasal fossa, where air is warmed and moistened for maximum oxygen uptake in the lungs and from there to be delivered via blood to the brain.

- **Orthognathic ('putting the jaw right') surgery**
If there is a dramatic mismatch between the relative sizes of the upper jaw and the lower jaw such that it is impossible to correct the bite with teeth extractions and braces alone, there is the third option of a surgical operation. This is done either to shorten, lengthen or otherwise change the shape of the lower jaw or, less commonly, to broaden the roof of the mouth, the palate.

Orthognathic procedures will aim to alter the shape of the jawbone in an attempt to match its appearance and size to that of the middle face. Such surgery presents a dramatic and sudden challenge to the biomechanics of the cranium, and this often takes place in adulthood when plasticity of the skull is diminished and the dura is unlikely to be able to reconcile such a drastic change. The mechanical conflict is too great and the outcome may be a fatigued and confused dural membrane system and consequent membrain disorder.

Sally

Sally, a 35-year-old computer analyst, walked into my practice some fifteen years ago hoping that I could help her with long-term spinal pain and sciatic pain going down into her left leg. The pains were debilitating and seemingly untreatable.

"I've seen consultants, physiotherapist, acupuncturists, energy worker, masseurs. You name them, I've seen them!" She would attend up to three or four different sessions with as many therapists a week and had done so for years. Osteopathy was next on the list to try. It was clear she wasn't holding out much hope. Her therapies had been costing her a fortune, but clearly so far she had failed to find a solution.

The pain in her spine and leg was only one of the reasons that Sally found life hard. She had also fallen out with her entire family, struggled socially and appeared to have no friends. Work was office-based but Sally complained about her workmates, who clearly found as much fault with her as she did with them. She was unsettled, angry, lonely and failing to thrive. In short, she was finding the world painful, hostile and disappointing.

The most significant detail in Sally's case history, as it unfolded, was that at the age of eighteen she had undergone orthognathic surgery: surgery to correct the jaw. There is a corrective procedure to adjust the size of the lower jawbone (the mandible) performed by a maxillofacial (jaw and face) surgeon. In Sally's case her lower jaw was protruding forward. This is a common trait which occurs when the lower face develops in childhood more than the middle face and carries the lower set of teeth forward of the upper set. The technical term is a Class 3 Skeletal. The operation is done mainly for cosmetic reasons but also to correct the way the upper and lower teeth meet together: the 'dental occlusion' or closing of the teeth.

My diagnosis on examining Sally was that her body had been trying to adapt to this abrupt structural change ever since she had

had the operation and the adaptation had proved too much for the dura to cope with. Her membrane system was fatigued, congested and ineffective (there were no pulls anywhere) and this was not just in her skull, it pervaded her whole body. The whole fascial system had effectively collapsed. Sally had little to no capacity to mechanically self-correct.

My biggest challenge was to dissuade Sally from seeing all her other therapists. She had become reliant on or addicted to treatment, perhaps because the practitioners were the only people from whom she received any kindness. Perhaps her quest for an effective therapy was a desperate search for emotional help, not just relief from physical pain. I persuaded her to see me, just me, and she came once every two weeks over a nine-month period.

Slowly, things improved. The nerve pain coming from her lower back gradually recovered but she still suffered intermittent lower back, neck and shoulder pain. However, throughout this time and up until the last time I saw Sally, when she had left her current job and was going to live elsewhere, I felt that I, also, had failed to help her. Pain flitted around her body. In my opinion her body was failing to organise a satisfactory compensation for the abrupt structural changes that had occurred when she underwent the dental surgery in her late teens.

Since that time, I have seen a number of patients who have had the same abrupt procedure to 'correct' the position of the jawbone. Each one has suffered, like Sally, with chronic musculoskeletal problems and psychological issues.

UNDERSTANDING THE RISKS OF ORTHOGNATHIC SURGERY

The operative procedure that Sally underwent as described above was traditionally done for medical reasons but increasingly is carried out for cosmetic effect. One would assume that a corrective procedure done largely for cosmetic reasons would be a fairly minor operation, the patient ending up with better looks and no post-operative consequences other than positive ones. YouTube is awash with upbeat faces beaming into their cameras, clearly delighted with the cosmetic effect of the operation.

On crossing paths with patients in my practice who have experienced facial surgery of this kind, I have found this picture of happier patients with problem-free experiences to be only a skin-deep scenario.

My experience with patients who have undergone this procedure is that the dural membrane system often cannot adapt to such an abrupt change and this reflects in long-term structural and mental conditions that are particularly difficult to treat, as seen in Sally. These conditions, again, are rarely if ever associated by either dentist or patient with the surgical procedure.

Over the years I have given numerous lectures at postgraduate level on the subject of the face. With each new cohort of students, I have asked whether any of them has had this procedure or know of patients, relatives or friends who have. The consensus, far more often than not, is: chronic musculoskeletal problems throughout the body and deep psychological issues.[43]

Knowing from clinical experience that any surgery on the skull can potentially impact on the dura and thus the brain and mental health, I have searched high and wide for research papers on the effect of orthognathic surgery on the long-term mental health of the patient. They are there, the research is done (by the medical profession that apparently unreservedly advocates this procedure) and the vast majority of these research papers suggest that clinical evidence supports an improved overall psychological state for patients post-operatively compared to pre-operatively.

There are rare cases where a link is made between a surgical intervention and subsequent declining mental health. This link is explained by suggesting the psychological issue, perhaps a psychosis, that developed after the intervention was somehow lying dormant in the patient all the time or was steroid-induced, a consequence of post-operative medication.[44, 45] Beyond the immediate post-operative discomfort (pain and swelling) the traumatic long-term physical impact of the procedure itself on mental health seems never to be questioned.

Eleanor

I met Eleanor about ten years ago, a wonderfully funny beautiful woman who collapsed a few months after the birth of her third child. It happened suddenly and unexpectedly. She was found in her kitchen, fallen to the floor, unable to move because she was so disabled by a feeling of utter powerlessness – both physical and mental.

Eleanor had started a well-known teeth alignment programme some weeks beforehand. The procedure involved the teeth being moved in stages. The aim was to arrange the teeth into a 'perfect' dental arc.

Eleanor had a plagiocephalic skull. It did not detract from her beauty in any way. It was an asymmetry visible, as is so often the case, only to those trained to look. She was exhausted from the recent birth of her third baby and looking after her family. Her whole system took the assault of the teeth alignment programme as the metaphorical final straw. Her body and mind gave up.

Luckily for us both, Eleanor was early on in the orthodontic process and was happy to try stopping the dental alignment programme, for a while at least. She recovered relatively quickly after stopping the programme. Without the constant pressure of the teeth alignment process, her plagiocephalic skull returned to its previous comfortable state. Eleanor no longer needs my intervention except for the most minor amount of support now and then.

Eleanor's was a classic case of membrain disorder diagnosed and corrected. Her dura and skull had long ago successfully adapted to her lifelong plagiocephaly, but at some cost; they were not adaptable to new changes. The tipping point came with the infliction of a low-grade, constant and conflicting force operating through her middle and lower face from the braces used in trying to straighten her teeth.

The irony is that those with asymmetrical skulls are, for that very reason, the most likely to have the cross bites, overbites, underbites and wonky teeth that dentists – and increasingly their patients – are so keen to straighten. This means that those with an already hard-worked brain housing are the most likely recipients of cosmetic orthodontic work impacting the skull. They will also be the least tolerant of the extra strain on their system.

The assault on Eleanor's brain housing affected her brain and thus her mental health in a particularly direct and dramatic way. Had she been referred to medical or mental health services, the collapse would almost certainly have been put down to factors such as recent childbirth and physical exhaustion. No one would even think to ask whether her dental work might have anything to do with it. The teeth straightening programme would no doubt have continued, and Eleanor's debilitating condition could have worsened.

The orthodontic procedure Eleanor received had an ongoing, low impact, but significant traumatic effect on the whole skull. The whole skull is the figurative box in which the brain sits – it is the environment of the central nervous system. Altering the environment alters the system.

BEING ALERT TO MEMBRAIN DISORDER

Many people reading this book who have been involved in an orthodontic intervention or orthognathic surgery, either personally or via their children, may have benefited from the procedure and experienced no side-effects. The skull has been impacted to some extent but the dural membrane has worked effectively to adapt to the changes in the skull and found a new way for the twenty-two bones to sit in a comfortable relationship with one another. However, in a proportion of such patients the dura, for one reason or another, will *not* have succeeded in restoring that comfortable relationship, especially where fixed retainers are creating a constant biomechanical strain on the whole cranial system which the dura cannot overcome.

The outcomes of such unresolved biomechanical conflicts are variable in terms of symptoms but may include mental health issues – a typical consequence of membrain disorder. Other symptoms include headaches, migraines, tinnitus, spinal pain, wrist and arm symptoms, poor energy, poor sleep and a host of other symptoms. The onset of these symptoms will have been insidious – meaning that they emerge gradually over time and are seldom attributed to the work done on the teeth or the retainers fixed in the mouth maintaining that perfect smile.

At present, neither dentists, oral and maxillofacial surgeons nor patients would think to associate these interventions with the gradual onset of mental and physical health problems. This possibility needs to be considered and appropriate studies need to be done so that both practitioners and patients can, with confidence, assess the risk to the long-term physical and mental health of both adults and children contemplating these procedures. Longer term studies are required; broader and more searching questions need to be asked

Most osteopaths trained in the cranial field will have practices awash with patients suffering from palpable distortions of an exhausted dural membrane system, one that has tried to autocorrect over years or even decades and failed. These patients often have a beautiful set of straight teeth, held firmly in place by permanently fixed retainers – but behind the perfect symmetry of the mouth sits an asymmetrical cranial base and vault. There is a mismatch here that cannot be reconciled. This was the case with Dido, the ballerina introduced at the beginning of this chapter.

It is a difficult task trying to tell a parent, who has probably spent thousands of pounds on top of endless after-school visits to the orthodontist, that the retainers maintaining a now perfect smile may be a contributing factor to their teenager's mental health problem. It is equally difficult trying to tell a 14-year-old girl who was so relieved to get those 'train tracks' off her teeth and the one good thing in her now depressed, OCD, anxiety-riddled life is a beautiful set of straight white teeth, that the retainers need to come off in order for her to feel good. It can be an impossible task. This again was the case with Dido.

A concern about the rising tide of dentistry-related membrain disorder is one of the main reasons for writing this book. What is happening to the delicate environment of the brain, behind the patient's face and behind that 'perfect' set of teeth is rarely, if ever, taken into consideration – before, during, or after an orthodontic intervention, at any age – by anyone.

A SOLUTION

An easy way to change this is for new parents to be made aware that they can search out an orthodontist who advocates expansion work and then start this at an early age. The current approach in the dental profession is to wait until most of the adult teeth have come through (about age 12) before referring a child to an orthodontist. Ideally they would refer to an orthodontist who specialised in the 'functional' approach at about 7 years of age.

An adult considering straightening their teeth for cosmetic effect could be made aware that it is not always an easy procedure without side-effects. On making a decision to go ahead it is important that the patient pays very close attention to general and mental health over the months during and after the procedure and is prepared to stop the procedure if anything 'feels' wrong.

Treatment and advice from a manual practitioner who understands membrain disorder is particularly useful alongside any orthodontic intervention, especially if there is a working relationship between the dentist and the manual practitioner.

There are, of course, medical conditions where an adult may be suffering with a severe malocclusion and associated jaw problems, headaches or spinal pain that require an orthodontic intervention which will ultimately be of benefit not only to the face but to the whole cranium, the whole person. The same applies to children. In these cases it is relatively straightforward to weigh the benefits against any possible side-effects.

The key point is that the biomechanics of the whole cranium should be considered in any orthodontic treatment plan, not just the specific issue of occlusion of the teeth and the desire to create a 'perfect' smile.

The increasing demand for a 'perfect' smile has led to a significant expansion in the amount of orthodontic work carried out for purely cosmetic reasons. Cosmetic dentistry is a major industry. According to the US website Business Wire, the global orthodontic consumables market was worth $5.2 billion in 2020 and is expected to more than double by 2027.[46] That's just the supplies!

The dental profession in the UK and elsewhere is governed by strict ethical guidelines but as a profession it is unaware of the impact of dental work on the skull and the potential consequences for mental health through membrain disorder.

SEVEN

A SYNOPSIS OF MEMBRAIN DISORDER

The concept of membrain health introduces the idea that there is a relationship between the state of the dural membrane and the behaviour of the brain. A poor relationship will result in membrain disorder. Membrain disorder can have an impact on mental health

AN UNDERSTANDING OF MEMBRAIN DISORDER

Abnormal housing of the brain can involve the bony skull, the underlying dural membrane, the irrigation system of the brain, or, most commonly, a combination of these factors.

Altered behaviour of the brain due to abnormal housing can manifest as a psychological issue. Where there is prolonged poor irrigation of an area of the brain due to membrain disorder this can create, sometimes over decades, a predisposition to early onset degenerative changes of the brain, including diseases such as CTE, Parkinson's and Alzheimer's.

It is in the patient's interest to understand when the membrain concept is relevant to their psychological state and whether they may be suffering from membrain disorder.

COMMON CAUSES OF MEMBRAIN DISORDER

1. TRAUMA

A common cause of membrain disorder would be a physical injury to the head or face. An injury can take many forms, whether a single strong blow, multiple repetitive knocks over years or other causes of long sustained pressure on the skull. Such incidents may either be regarded as insignificant or long forgotten, or the patient remembers the injury but never imagines it has anything to do with their current depression or disturbed thoughts and emotions.

a. Birth

For the vast majority of us, being born is probably the biggest trauma that our heads have ever experienced (figure 20). It is the dura, the tough tadpole-shaped container – not the bony skull as one might expect – that really copes with the pressures and twists imposed on the head as it passes down the birth canal. The dura, through its design, has the capacity to withstand huge forces via what is called *tensegrity*. Any architect or physicist will concur that tensile structures arranged in certain configurations create stable forms able to withstand huge and varied external forces. The human spine itself maintains its form not as a consequence of the vertebrae that sit one on top of another but by tensile forces that come from the arrangement of soft tissue structures such as the ligaments which have evolved to exist in very particular configurations.[47, 48]

The dural membrane is a three-dimensional arrangement which, combined with the orientation of its fibres, maintains strength and stability but also flexibility to the entire head complex (figure 21). The dura is able to withstand the compressions and rotational and sideway forces to the skull that are part of the birth process. The dura, the 'tough mother of the brain', really is an extraordinary parent who has received little to no attention (until now)!

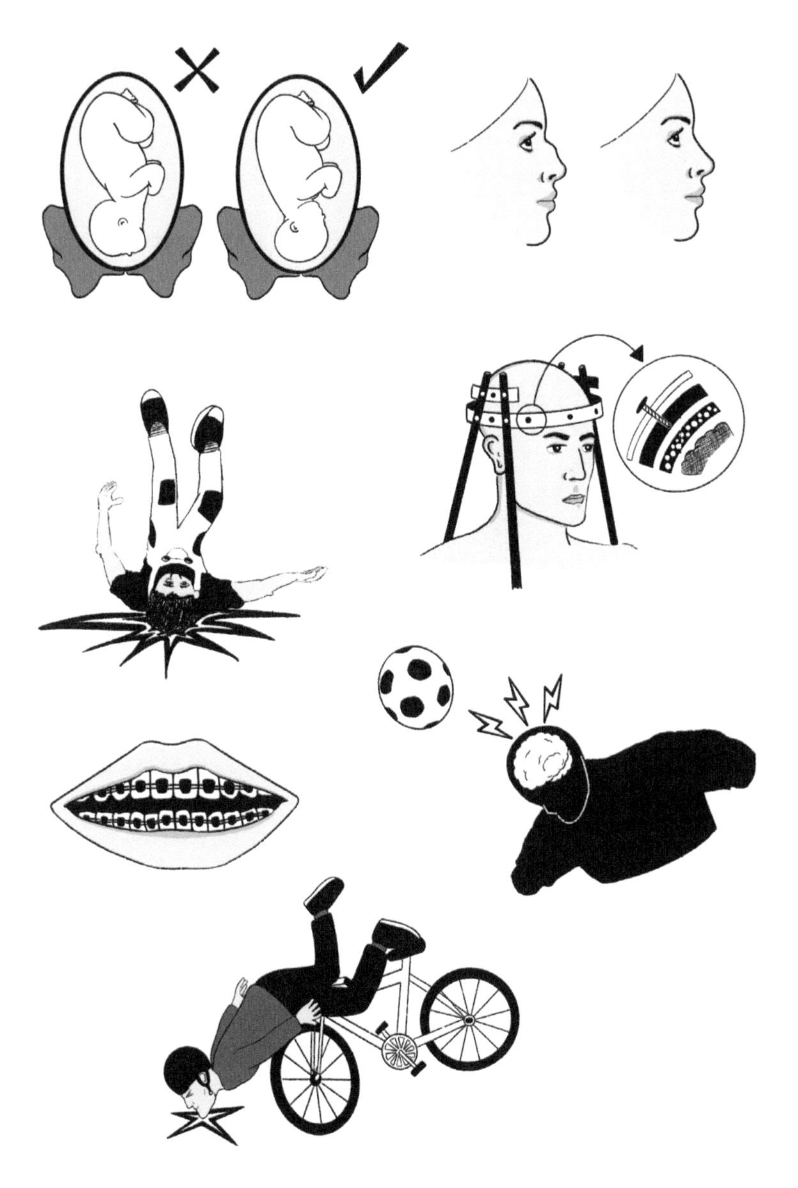

Figure 20. Different types of head trauma

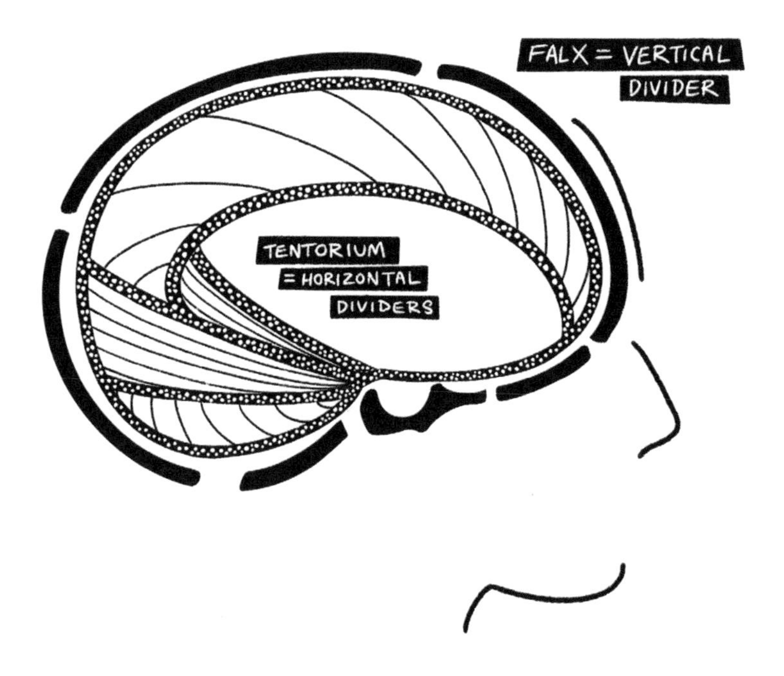

Figure 21. Side view of the vertical and horizontal dividers of the dura. Together they create a three-dimensional flexible structure. This, combined with the anchor points of attachment onto the bones, provides tensegrity to the whole cranial system.

It is helpful when patients know about their birth and whether it was easy or traumatic, quick or prolonged. The birth may have involved forceps, or a suction cup on the head, or an emergency caesarean. This does not mean that these medical processes caused any injury; it reveals that the baby was stuck at some point in the birth canal, probably because the head was in the wrong position (figure 20). When this happens, a part of the skull that hasn't been designed to withstand the forces of labour takes the trauma of the birth. Being a twin or a triplet can also create complications. Research linking complications of delivery and schizophrenia suggests that this is a consequence of anoxia (a loss of oxygen to the brain) during the birthing process rather than trauma to the skull and unresolved legacies in the dural membrane system.[49]

Giving birth involves two; the mother as well as the baby will experience physical trauma during childbirth and it is worth mentioning that post-natal depression in the mother can be linked to membrain disorder. This is because the tail of the tadpole-shaped dural membrane is connected at its lowest point to the inner surface of the pelvis. Unresolved trauma to the pelvis can create a 'dragging-down' effect on the entire dural membrane system. This is a physical condition, potentially affecting the mental health of the mother – a condition that can be diagnosed and treated.

b. Accidental head trauma – childhood

A common cause of head trauma for a baby, besides birth, is being dropped accidentally or, for example, propelling themselves off the changing mat. It happens!

In older children, obvious causes might be falling off climbing frames, trampolines, walls, bikes or out of trees.

c. Abusive head trauma – childhood

There is a 'blind spot' that permeates studies into mental health and child abuse that is specifically physical – a child who is hit or shaken. Scientific research papers looking into childhood abuse and later psychological issues often don't differentiate between emotional and physical abuse.

It is not hard to discover why physical violence is not separated out from other forms of abuse, on looking at the way the term 'child abuse' is defined. There is no single definition of child abuse, but that supplied by the World Health Organization is perhaps the most comprehensive and influential among authors of research papers. It runs:

> [Child abuse is] *all forms of physical and/or emotional ill-treatment, sexual abuse, neglect or negligent treatment or commercial or other exploitation, resulting in actual or potential harm to the child's health, survival, development or dignity in the context of a relationship of responsibility, trust or power.*[50]

This WHO definition is no doubt helpful in identifying a global mental health issue caused by the mistreatment of children that demands attention. However, using this definition as a starting point for research into mental health means lumping "all forms of physical and/or emotional" abuse together. It is obvious that the idea of lasting but undiagnosed physical damage to certain children may easily be neglected.

So long as membrain disorder remains absent from global consciousness, no one will look for it as a *physical* condition in those who have suffered as children. Specific injuries caused by physical abuse, particularly if a child was hit in the head and face, may be a significant contributor to their subsequent and often long-lasting psychological issues. The same is true for adults who have experienced abuse of a physical nature.

d. Repetitive head trauma – childhood and adult

As discussed in chapter 2, certain contact sports played regularly will result in repeated low-grade impacts to the head. There are now well-documented statistical links between repetitive head trauma, mental health problems and early onset brain disease in boxers, footballers, rugby players and the like. The authorities are well aware of the dangers, but unaware of how knocks on the skull can cause mental health problems or why this should lead later to Parkinson's, Alzheimer's and other brain diseases. Short of banning these sports, all they can do is impose health and safety restrictions.

By approaching the issue from the point of view of membrain disorder, it can be seen that the initial damage from the type of repetitive impacts so often received in contact sports is not to the brain directly, but to the housing of the brain, i.e. the skull, the dura and the fluids that surround or nourish the brain. Mood swings and behavioural changes in young sports people may be early warning signs. These may also indicate a predisposition to early-onset degenerative changes to the brain caused by poor irrigation (for example limiting the brain's blood supply) over long periods of time. The brain will start to change not just its behaviour, but also eventually its structure if it lives in a stressful environment for too long. This can be remedied if diagnosed and treated in time.

2. *THE TEETH*

General consensus does not link the eruption of new teeth nor ongoing teeth or occlusal problems through life with altered brain function, thus affecting thoughts and behaviour. The configuration of the middle and lower face continues to change throughout the whole of our life with first teeth erupting, milk teeth being replaced with permanent teeth and eventual loss of some or all of the permanent teeth. The vault and base of the skull are constantly adapting to these changes over the years and decades.

a. Infant teething

Concerned parents sometimes bring their young children with behavioural problems that have developed out of the blue. These cases provide a very simple example of how what is happening to the teeth can affect the emotions and the general health of that person – contrary to what most might think!

The very first thing to do in such a situation is see if the child has any new teeth coming through. The classic case is when a small child, normally aged between one and a half and two years old, starts biting their little friends – all totally out of character. This tends to happen as the canines or eye teeth start coming through. Although it seems alarming, this is a phase that can be explained in evolutionary terms. Canines are killer teeth. Biting is instinctive behaviour, it is all very transient and the biting will settle once the canine teeth have fully come through.

At the age of about six, a child will still have most of his or her milk teeth, but behind the scenes all the big teeth are there, embedded in the bone and all jostling for position with very little space. It is a chaotic situation that can easily set off the dural membrane system and cause minor havoc in the skull. The child may be inattentive in class, suffering from disturbed sleep or upsetting the family with their behaviour. Very often this stage of teeth development also generates ear problems. These are part of growing up. It is possible to reassure the parents by explaining the cause, but very little can be done for the child, and time is the healer. Eventually the new teeth will find their place, the tadpole-shaped dura will resume its normal state, the brain will be comfortable once again and the child's behaviour will revert to normal. These examples show how the skull and the underlying membrane system that house the brain act as a responsive living environment that influences the behaviour of the brain, including disturbed thoughts, emotions and behaviour.

The other big troublemakers are the wisdom teeth (the big

molar teeth at the very back) that emerge around the age of eighteen. These teeth are often short of space, causing them to lie at odd angles, sometimes trapped in the bone but still trying to find a route to cut through the gum. This can create abnormal and unequal forces through the jawbone and backwards into the skull. Removing the wisdom teeth, as is often done, requires varying degrees of trauma giving the dura a lot to take care of.

b. Orthodontics

As described previously in chapter 6, membrain disorder can arise particularly from orthodontic work. Although the front part of the skull, the 'face', does not house the brain, it has a very intimate relationship with the other two parts of the skull, the cranial 'base' and the 'vault', and these two directly house the brain. Any deliberate alteration to the way the teeth meet will affect the relationship between the middle and lower face and this will impact backwards into the whole skull, affecting bony relationships that the dura then has to work to reconcile, successfully or not.

c. General dentistry

Moving on through the decades, any dental intervention in adulthood can be traumatic: a difficult tooth extraction, hours in the dentist chair having a root canal treatment, undergoing a dental implant and – increasingly often nowadays – major cosmetic work. Just remaining with jaws widely apart for a long period of time under stressful circumstances can create a problem for the skull. Then there is the trauma of the procedure itself. The dental work may involve force such as the difficult removal of a tooth with pliers or the drilling required for a root canal treatment. All can have an impact on the skull. Dental bridges or plates which spread across a number of teeth can have the same effects as the retainers fixed in children. People rarely, if ever, attribute the onset of an episode of depression or other mental health problems to their recent, or even long-past, trip to the dentist.

3. MEDICAL TREATMENTS

a. Head, facial and oral surgery

Any type of surgical intervention to the head, face or jaw can trigger membrain disorder. Examples would be a cosmetic nose operation, surgery to the jaw or a sinus operation.

All surgical procedures on the different parts of the skull can have a significant influence on the housing and thus the behaviour of the brain and an impact on psychological health.

b. Spine fractures and the 'halo brace'

The halo brace is a medical contraption used to immobilise the neck if there has been a fracture to the upper part of the spine. Certain halo braces remain fixed onto the patient via a metal ring (the 'halo') that circles the skull. The halo is held by pins screwed directly into the skull. It may be several months before the neck is considered to be stable and the halo brace is removed.

In the best case scenario, not only the neck bones but also the nerves will have healed and a patient will leave hospital seemingly cured. But what if those pins, now removed, that had been fixed into the patient's skull, have compressed the individual bones of the cranial vault, to the point that the dura cannot manage to return the delicate bones of the skull to their normal state? This could result in membrain disorder and a patient who leaves the hospital, seemingly cured, dealing then or later with a debilitating depression which has no apparent cause.

The halo brace may be necessary to hold the head in position but the possible consequences for mental health should be anticipated and addressed if they occur. Patients who have been fitted with a halo brace should be alert to the possibility of mental health consequences and examined for membrain disorder once the brace is removed so that potentially lasting damage to the skull can receive preventive treatment at an early stage.[51]

HEAD TRAUMA AND PTSD

There are many cases of people suffering from historical emotionally traumatic events that can lead to post-traumatic stress disorder (PTSD).

Some of these historical events are entirely emotionally based, for example the death of a loved one or being an observer of a shocking or horrifying event. Alternatively some of these historical events may involve being subjected to a physical trauma as well as an emotional assault such as being tortured, injured in battle or being mugged.

There have been many scientific studies into the links between violent physical assaults on both children and adults and the victims' short-term and long-term mental health. Questions raised in the research projects presuppose that the mental health problems of the victim stem entirely from some mental 'memory' or 'trace' of the emotional impact of being attacked, not from the physical impact itself.[52]

The concept of membrain health suggests that it is important to be alert not just to the emotional impact of the event at the time but also to any physical trauma (especially a head injury) that could have impacted the biomechanics of the skull and left an invisible but very real legacy of abnormality in the brain's housing which contributes to the enduring symptoms of PTSD. It is notable that some victims suffer from PTSD and others do not – a disparity usually attributed to individual mental resilience,[53] but in some cases it could be explained by the dura's success or lack of it in resolving a physical injury to the skull.

This lack of interest in the physical body would seem extraordinary if the researchers were physicians, but of course research into PTSD is located in the field of mental health and it focuses on patients who present with ongoing psychological problems, usually long after the physical injuries have – apparently – healed. This disregard of the patient's body is evident very early on in research papers on PTSD and the like where it quickly becomes obvious that little or no attention is being paid to exactly how the victims were attacked, exactly where on their body they received physical blows, and what were the nature and frequency of those blows.

PROFESSIONAL DIAGNOSIS OF MEMBRAIN DISORDER

An appropriately trained manual therapist in the cranial field would be able to diagnose membrain disorder and, most importantly, treat it. 'Appropriately trained' means they would have acquired a thorough anatomical knowledge of the skull, its individual bones, the dura, the fluid systems of the brain and the brain itself. They would also need advanced palpatory skills and the ability to perform balanced membranous tension (BMT), the 'indirect' treatment approach to influencing the dura discussed in chapter 4.

Diagnosis is achieved by a combination of: (1) visual observation – looking for signs of plagiocephaly, scars on the face or chin; (2) interview – a thorough case history, taking account of all physical injuries, medical and dental interventions, and finally; (3) palpation – feeling and 'listening' to the body through the hands, remembering that the membranes, including the dura, tell a story.

TREATMENT OF MEMBRAIN DISORDER

If this combination of approaches indicates that membrain disorder is a contributory factor to the patient's mental health, an 'indirect' BMT (Balanced Membranous Tension) approach can be used in an attempt to resolve the problem. This is the method that supports the dura in what it is already trying to do, helping to restore things to a comfortable state. It is a 'listening', caring, gentle and highly effective approach, based on simple but little-known physical principles and with far reaching consequences. As with everything there are degrees of success in any medical intervention and the degree of success is dependent on many factors, as shown in the case studies. Whatever the degree of success, it will represent a significant step in the right direction towards a recovery – and sometimes it is a leap.

If it is not possible to gain any information from palpating the membrane system then there is probably no story to tell, at least as far as the manual therapist is concerned. This does not mean the patient does not have a problem, only that its cause (social, emotional, genetic, chemical, etc.) falls outside the remit and treatment capabilities of the manual therapist.

In this case, the role of the manual practitioner is to recognise that the patient is struggling psychologically but the origin of that disorder is not the physical housing of the central nervous system. In other words, membrain disorder is not a cause of the mental health issue. If the practitioner is able have an idea what the origin might be, at what 'dimension' that patient is struggling, then he or she can provide the invaluable service of referring the patient on – and in the right direction.

A BROADER DIAGNOSIS OF MENTAL HEALTH PROBLEMS

The mention of the 'dimension' at which a psychological problem originates leads on to the second part of this book – a broader perspective on how to diagnose and then care for mental health patients that differs from the current system. It is an approach that places the membrain health concept in context with all the other important and varied considerations that come into play when facing a patient in deep psychological distress.

Oliver Kamm in his book *Mending the Mind* tries to consider the possible causes for depression but acknowledges that research remains inconclusive. He is however sure of one thing: that depression is a "disorder of a physical organ, and the most complex one we have: the brain."[54] That insight fits well with the story so far about membrain health. But the brain, too, is just one dimension of the complex human biological system. Certainly the brain is involved in depression, but where does the problem originate?

A disorder causing a mental health problem such as depression can originate from any of a number of dimensions, from the macro dimension of the individual and his or her social circumstances all the way down to the micro dimension of the neurotransmitters, the unseen biomolecular level. Of course, because of the interrelationship between the different dimensions the brain will inevitably be involved but it is the identification of the *dimensional origin* of the disorder that is the key to understanding a patient's individual condition. And understanding the origin helps the practitioner to understand the best therapeutic approach.

A patient's individual condition is not to be confused with its label. A label such as 'depression' describes a collection of symptoms, not their cause, or causes. Part Two of this book explores the different dimensions at which mental health problems with the same label can originate within the complex human biological system, locating membrain disorder in a broader context and proposing a different approach to the diagnosis – and hence treatment – of mental health conditions.

PART TWO

COMPLEXITY AND MENTAL HEALTH: THE DIMENSIONAL MODEL

EIGHT

A NEW APPROACH TO MENTAL HEALTH DIAGNOSIS

When it comes to mental illness, how, and by whom, is a mental health diagnosis arrived at within modern Western society? There are no blood tests or MRI scans performed. There are no visible marks of disease to be observed by the doctor similar to a rash in chickenpox or a swollen joint in arthritis. Diagnosis in the mental health field is based purely on analysis of symptoms as reported by the patient and from observed behaviour. When it comes to the most common mental health issues such as depression or anxiety, the symptoms are subjective to the patient and the patient is expected to describe their condition in words or may be asked to fill out one of a variety of multiple-choice questionnaires that have been designed to 'measure' depression or anxiety or other labelled mental conditions.[55,56]

There is an irony here. Each person is inherently of two minds. The right hemisphere of our brain has been shown to hold a closer association with the emotional centres and yet the right hemisphere has no verbal representative. Speech is formulated in 'Broca's area' which is located in the left hemisphere of the brain. Trying to diagnose a patient's mental health problems by asking them to explain verbally the symptoms that they feel or to fill out a multiple-choice questionnaire (engaging the left hemisphere) about their feelings – where brain activity is focused in the right hemisphere to the exclusion of the left hemisphere – is fundamentally flawed.[57]

The next stage of diagnosis involves what is called the *Diagnostic and Statistical Manual of Mental Disorders* (DSM) first produced in the early 1950s and now in its fifth edition.[58] DSM-5 lists pre-defined groups of symptoms which are the criteria for identifying a diagnostic label. The diagnostic label that is picked out of the manual will influence the treatment prescribed, commonly a psychotropic drug. In a positive case scenario the drug helps; in a harmless case scenario the drug has no positive nor negative impact – it makes no difference. In a negative case scenario the named psychological condition gets worse and iatrogenic (treatment-caused) side-effects of the drugs add to the problem. In a worst-case scenario the outcome is dire and the drugs lead to a severe and sometimes sudden deterioration in the psychological state of the patient.

The current system that embraces DSM-5 is widely criticised, even by some who are trained and work within it. However, it is a system that is entrenched; it represents a mindset that has become established. Health professionals, medical researchers, medical insurance companies and drug companies rely on this system. Equally the patient also relies on it. Within Western culture someone who is unwell expects to be offered a named diagnosis or label for any physical or mental health condition. To explain a *cause* to a patient does not satisfy their expectation of receiving a *label* for their condition.

Mental health problems are escalating in the UK and elsewhere and the system in place is generally recognised to be unsatisfactory.[59, 60]

THE LABEL

A new and different way of describing a mental health condition that avoids a single label is offered by the American psychiatrist Steven Buser, author of *DSM-5 Insanely Simplified.*

Buser describes eight 'primary spectrums' of psychiatry (figures 22–29) as follows:

The Depression Spectrum

(How much SORROW do you hold?)

Ranges from *shallow* and *indifferent* (problematic) to *deep despair* and *hopelessness* (problematic). Middle range would be *empathic* and *caring* (non-problematic).

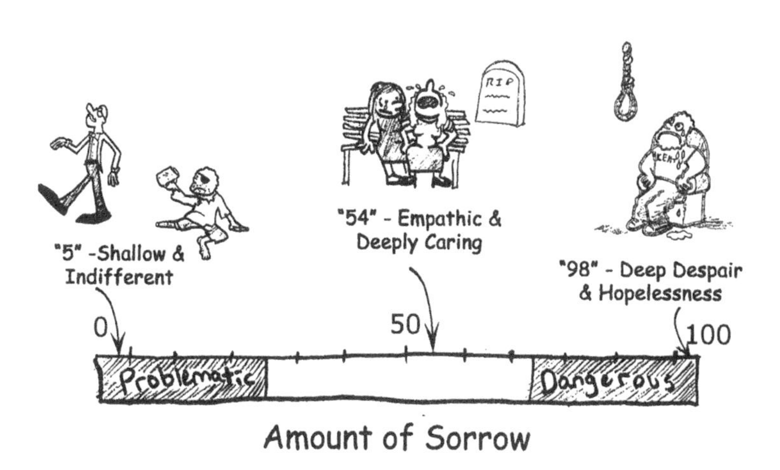

Figure 22. Depression spectrum.

Figures 22–29 reproduced by permission of Chiron Press.

The Mania Spectrum

(How much CREATIVITY do you have?)

Ranges from *no imagination* and *no get up and go* to *full mania* (both problematic). Middle range would be *fun party person* and *creative* (non-problematic).

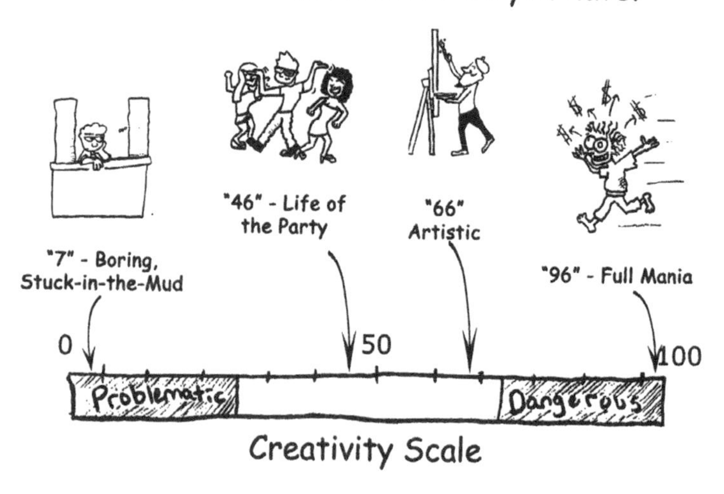

Figure 23. Mania spectrum

The Anxiety Spectrum

(How much VIGILANCE do you have?)

Ranges from *reckless* to *fear, anxiety* and *panic* (both problematic). Middle range would be *robustly enjoying life* (non-problematic)

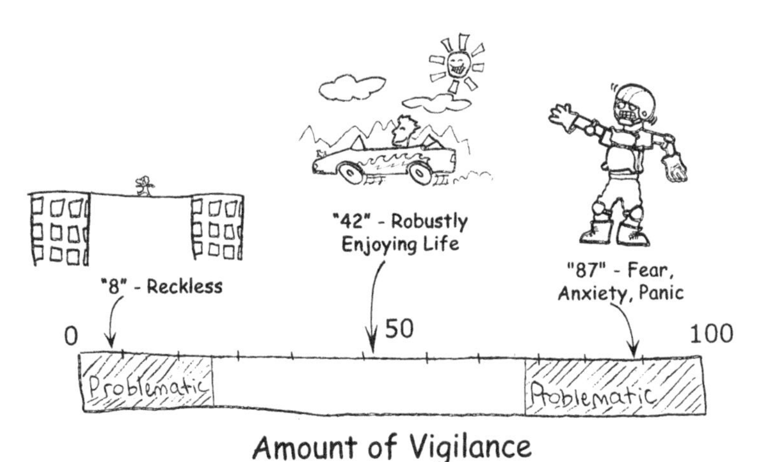

Figure 24. Anxiety spectrum

The Psychosis Spectrum

(How strong are your DREAMS and VISIONS?)

Ranges from *boring and uninspired* to *visions that have broken through reality into psychosis* (both problematic). Middle range would be *inspired and vision-filled* (non-problematic).

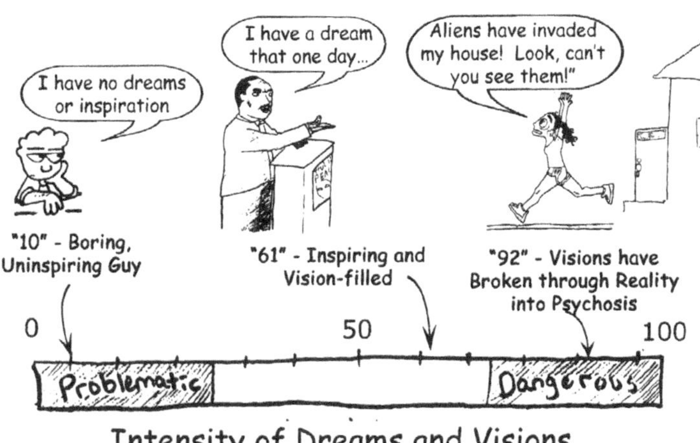

Figure 25. Psychosis spectrum

The Focus Spectrum

(How much FOCUS do you have?)

It can range from *can't sit still and focus* (ADHD type symptoms) to *obsessive compulsive disorder* (OCD) (both problematic). Middle range would be *healthy attention* (non-problematic).

Attention Deficit Disorder (ADHD)
vs. Obsessive Compulsive Disorder (OCD)
"How much FOCUS do you have?"

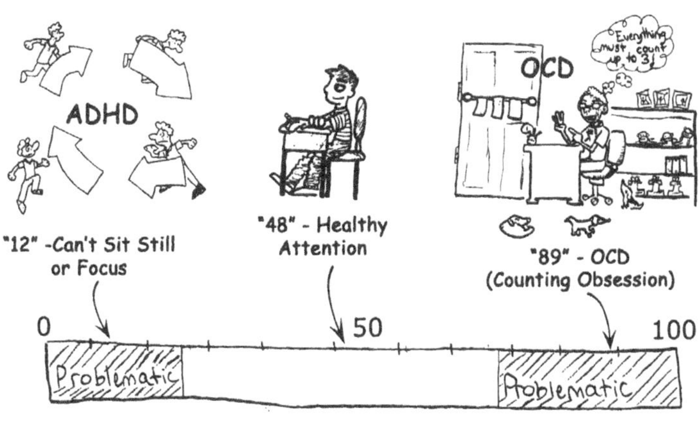

Figure 26. Focus spectrum

The Substance Abuse Spectrum

(How much PLEASURE do you seek?)

It can range from an *ascetic monk with no possessions* to *someone who parties all night with multiple drug addictions* (both problematic). Middle range would be *healthy enjoyment of wine and song* (non-problematic).

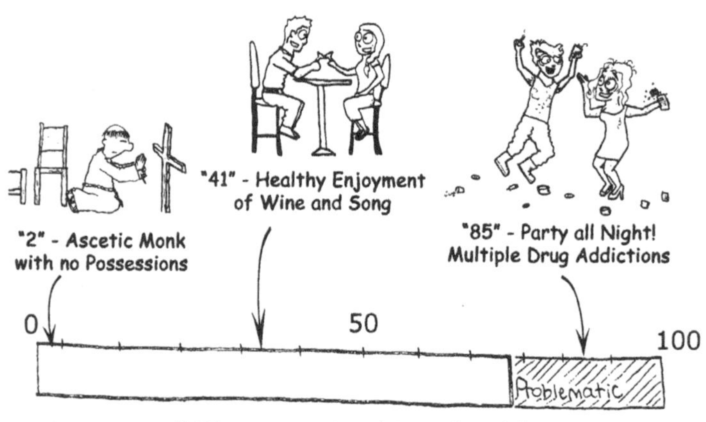

Figure 27. Substance abuse spectrum

The Autism Spectrum

(How CONNECTED TO OTHERS are you?)

It can range from *severe autism* to *severe co-dependency* (both problematic). Middle range would be *healthy friendships* (non-problematic).

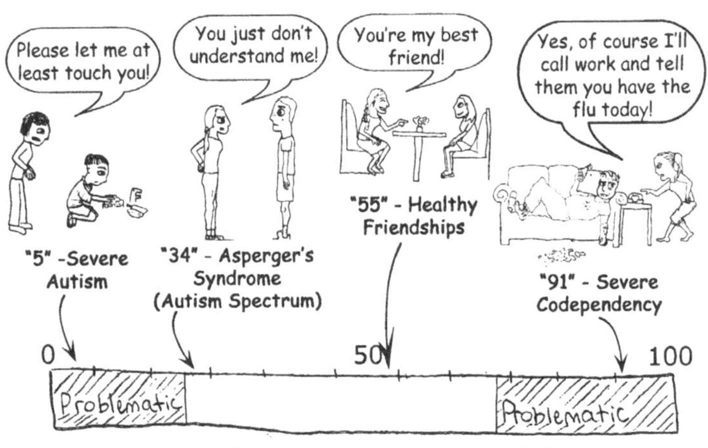

Figure 28. Autism spectrum

The Personality Spectrum

(How much BLAME do you cast?)

It can range from *taking all the blame oneself* to *always finding the blame to be with others* (both problematic). Middle range would be *a healthy respect for others and good boundaries* (non-problematic).

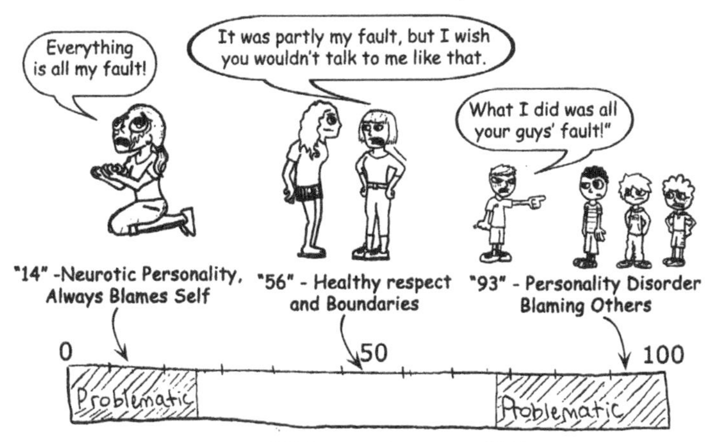

Figure 29. Personality spectrum

Buser writes:

> *Within each of these categories ['depression', 'mania', 'anxiety', etc.] there exists a spectrum. At the extremes of the spectrums problems emerge. The middle ranges of these spectrums are preferable. The extreme ranges, where symptoms of mental illness appear, tend to interfere with life....*
>
> *The middle of each spectrum is a zone of 'healthy functioning'. The power of this spectrum approach is that clinicians no longer must fit patients into either a category of 'healthy' or 'disordered'. Instead, gradations along a spectrum allow for more varied, nuanced understanding of the individual.*
>
> *The question facing clinicians now becomes not "does a person have bipolar disorder or not," but rather "how much bipolarity does a person have?" Everyone has some degree of bipolarity, for example, when overtaken by a surge of creativity, artistry, spontaneity, energy, sociability, talkativeness, and excitement. It is only when these features are 'out of control' or produce negative consequences that a person enters the realm of what DSM-5 considers a 'disorder'.*[61]

It is genius.

Buser describes how everybody falls somewhere along each of these eight spectrums and fluctuates along them constantly, hopefully maintaining themselves within the middle ranges. Just this idea takes the shame away from psychological illness. It also helps us accept the fact that everyone at stages in their life will struggle with their mental health and this is entirely normal.

If a patient is struggling mentally, rather than give them a label one can instead identify on which of the eight spectrums they are experiencing problems.

CAUSATIVE FACTORS

Once the concept of fluctuations along multiple spectrums of mental health is grasped, the next stage is to understand the *causative factors* that tip a person to an extreme end of one or more of these spectrums, such that they cannot recover. Day to day, week to week and year to year the fluctuations and the success in maintaining a balance within each category will be influenced by both biological factors and psychosocial factors. Yet, whilst psychosocial factors feature strongly in many a discussion around mental health problems, biological factors do not.

It is the causative factors that need to be identified and the causative factors that need to be addressed (by the relevant therapist) to enable a restoration of balance, such that the patient can move back towards the middle range on the spectrum(s).

In order to understand the range of causative factors systematically it is time to introduce complexity – albeit decomplexified!

NINE

COMPLEXITY*

In 2000, Stephen Hawking, in response to a question about the way that science is developing, replied: "*I think the next century will be the century of complexity.*"[62] He was pointing towards some increasingly important scientific ideas emerging in the 1980s and 1990s that allow us to find order within highly complex and interconnected systems. These include not only the weather, traffic movement, the stock market and ecosystems[63] but also digital systems and biological systems. It is the application of complexity thinking to biological systems that is of interest here. The human being is a biological system. The brain is a biological system. The nerve cell is a biological system. The 'mind' emerges from these biological systems interacting with one another and with their respective environments.

Like so many fields, the understanding of complexity (commonly referred to as general systems theory or GST) has become highly intellectualised and as a consequence rather

* This chapter draws on the teaching of Max Girardin and Jean-Paul Hoeppner (see Acknowledgments).

inaccessible to those non-academics picking up books or scientific articles on the subject. But as Stephen Lewin explains in his book *Complexity: Life at the Edge of Chaos*, the theory is based on simple principles. By applying these simple principles in the field of health a rationale emerges that can be applied to the understanding of health and disease. This is the foundation of the 'biopsychosocial model' introduced by George Engel in 1977.[64] Engel proposed that psychological and social factors should be considered alongside biological factors in the understanding and diagnosis of illness. It is a model that has been both embraced and criticised over the decades but it has stood the test of time.[65, 66]

In this second part of the book, the emphasis is on complexity and mental health *diagnosis*. Attention is drawn towards the different biological dimensions (as well as the psychological and social dimensions) that can be the *cause* of psychological problems.

CHRONOLOGY AND TIME

Chronology is an aspect of complexity; it is the dimension of time. Chronology here refers to the sequential order in which systems form; what came first, then second, then third, etc.

Chronology exists in nature and can be observed in the evolution of life over billions of years from the earliest and simplest elements to the latest and most sophisticated forms of life.

Chronology can equally be observed in human embryology, the step-by-step development of each individual human from single fertilized cell to new-born baby.

The two are entirely different processes but both follow a sequential order over time, a chronology.

COMPLEXITY

Complexity theory posits that as chronological layers cumulate, so does the level of complexity. Parts come together to form a system and then that system, in turn, combines with other systems to become part of a new, more complex system.

SYSTEM

A system can be defined as anything that is composed of parts that organise themselves into a particular configuration in space and can maintain that configuration over a period of time.

At the start of the evolution of our universe there was the atom, a complex system of subatomic particles. The behaviour of that atom was governed by natural laws of attraction determining the the ability of the atom to self-maintain within its environment.[67] Atoms combined to form molecules, molecules to form organic molecules. Then came the advent of life. Organic molecules combined with water to form cells.

BIOLOGICAL COMPLEXITY AND DIMENSIONS

A Russian doll comprising six dolls, one within another, can provide a visual analogy representing the human biological and social systems occupying different dimensions of complexity (figure 30).

Each dimension represents a jump up in complexity as systems from the dimensions 'below' organise themselves to become parts of a new more complex system in the dimension 'above'. Cells aggregate in a particular configuration to form multicellular tissues, different multicellular tissues aggregate in a particular configuration to form organs and body systems. Organs and body systems exist in a particular configuration to form an individual and those individuals exist in social groups.

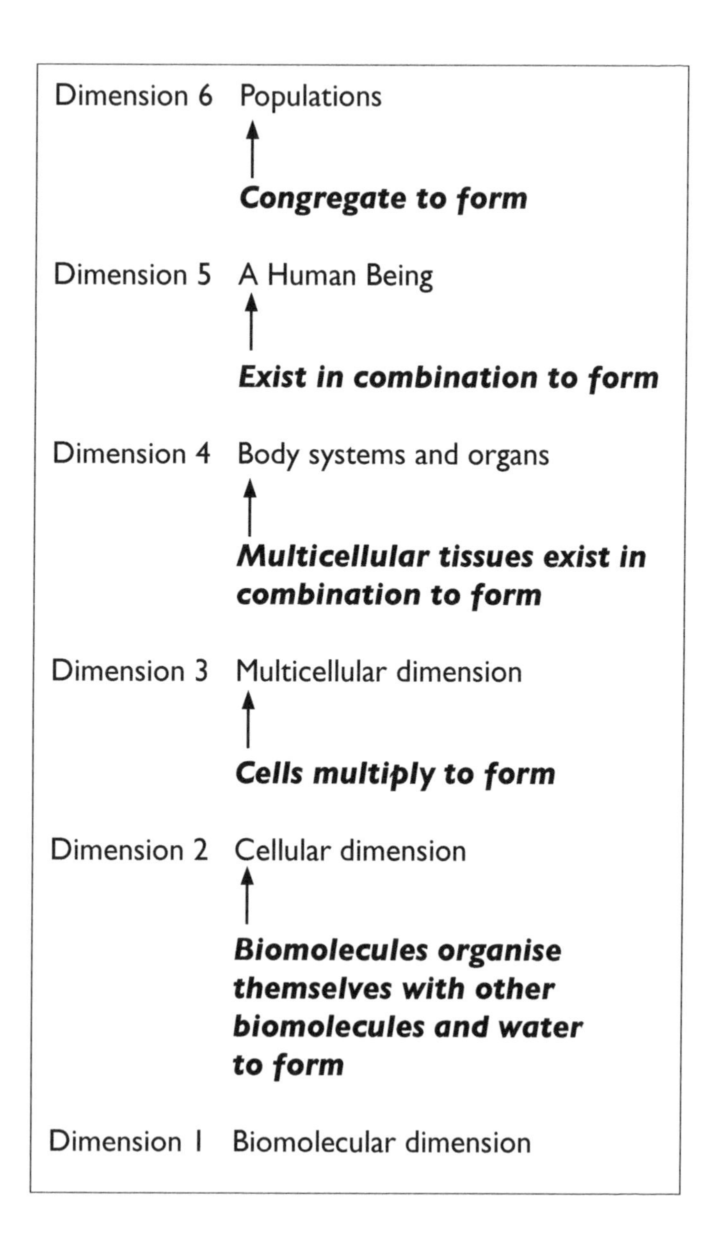
Dimension 6
Populations
Congregate to form
Dimension 5
A Human Being
Exist in combination to form
Dimension 4
Body systems and organs
Multicellular tissues exist in combination to form
Dimension 3
Multicellular dimension
Cells multiply to form
Dimension 2
Cellular dimension
Biomolecules organise themselves with other biomolecules and water to form
Dimension 1
Biomolecular dimension

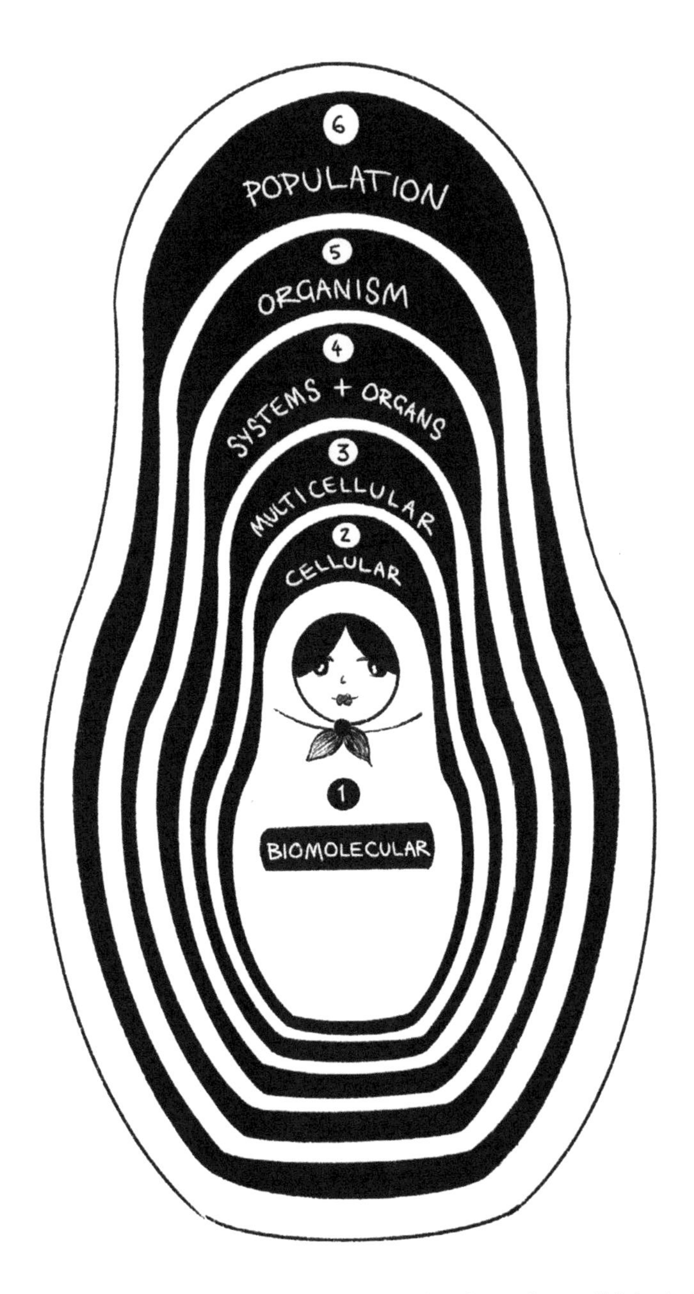

Figure 30. EVOLUTION represented in the chronology of biological systems

SELF-MAINTENANCE OF A COMPLEX SYSTEM

It is through forces of attraction and repulsion that a system will self-organise to create a form. Once a balance is established between the parts of any system, the forces operating among the parts will allow the system to self-maintain in that particular configuration over time – and this ability is reliant upon environmental conditions. If something from outside changes and, as a consequence of this change, there is a new stress on the system, it may have to adapt. There may be a shifting of the parts, but the outward appearance of the form remains unchanged; however its *behaviour* has changed. If on the other hand the forces exerted by the environment of a system change to such an extent that the system cannot maintain itself, the *form* will change. The system will either break down into its component parts – a jump down in complexity – or it will combine with another system to become a more resilient but more complex system – a jump up in complexity.

The self-maintenance of a system is a natural phenomenon. The ability of a system to self-maintain in a particular form is reliant on that system's environment.

SELF-MAINTENANCE OF A BIOLOGICAL SYSTEM (A COMPLEX ADAPTIVE SYSTEM)

Each dimension within a complex biological system is behaving according to natural laws.

Each dimension is either succeeding in maintaining itself (normal behaviour), adapting to maintain itself (altered behaviour) or failing (structural change).

An alternative way of thinking about health and disease is to identify the dimension at which a biological system is under stress and then to understand whether the consequence of that stress is simply an adaptive change in *behaviour* at that level (a 'pre-pathological' change) or whether there has been a radical *structural* reorganisation (a 'pathological' change).

This distinction is important because a pre-pathological change is reversible while a pathological change is not. This has a huge impact on choice of therapist, on where treatment is directed, and on the long-term prognosis for a patient.

In a pathological change (i.e. where there has been structural reorganisation) two things can happen. The system may have broken down to its component parts or it may have combined with another system to make a more complex system that is more robust. In medical terms the dissolution of the system into its component parts would be for example a degenerative condition such as CTE (Chronic Traumatic Encephalopathy) while increased complexity would be for example a cancerous growth.

THE ENVIRONMENT

The 'environment' of a system can take many forms.

Imagine a husband and wife (the couple is the system), both from happy backgrounds, both gainfully employed, nice house, well-balanced children and a good life. Their environment – comprising all these factors – is a stabilising force. If the environment changes – for example they lose their nice home in the midst of a financial crisis – the existing relationship between husband and wife will be challenged. If they can adapt their behaviour to their new financial situation then their relationship will survive.

Or consider a motorway full of traffic (the motorway traffic is the system), the drivers self-organising in lanes according to speed, responding to weather conditions and to roadwork signs that tell them to slow down for a while. They adjust their behaviour responsibly, adapting to environmental conditions and the overall traffic system is maintained.

A system responding to its environment in order to maintain itself is a natural phenomenon, and that responding is a form of *behaviour*.

However, a change in behaviour may not be sufficient to maintain a system. Take for example a forest (the forest is the system) that grows strongly over hundreds of years against a prevailing wind. It can withstand huge forces from the usual direction of the wind, but if one day a storm should come from a different direction, trees will fall. The form of the forest will alter as it is unable to adapt successfully to this extreme change in environmental conditions. A forest overwhelmed by changing environmental conditions has failed to maintain its structure, has decomplexified – and there are fewer trees in the forest – or perhaps no forest at all.

The effect of an environment on a system is an example of the 'outside-inside' phenomenon discussed in chapter 2. Sick building syndrome was used as an analogy to illustrate how abnormal housing of the brain represents a challenging environment that will inevitably influence the behaviour of the brain.

EMERGENT BEHAVIOUR

Each step up in the level of complexity of a system is marked by what is called 'emergence', or 'emergent behaviour'. This is where the properties of the more complex system arising from interaction in the dimension below are new and different from the properties of the individual components.

One very simple example of this is water. Water has a range of extraordinary (emergent) properties that bear no resemblance to the properties of hydrogen (H) or oxygen (O) of which it is composed. Hydrogen and oxygen have their own individual behaviours, but where combined they become water, a substance at a higher level of complexity whose behaviour is quite different from that of oxygen or hydrogen alone. All three behaviours exist within the space of the water; the hydrogen atoms behave as hydrogen atoms, the oxygen atoms behave as oxygen atoms and the water molecules behave as water molecules (1 behaviour + 1 behaviour = 3 behaviours).

Another example would be genetic modification of food –

genetic engineering. If unrelated genes are spliced together the behaviour of a resulting life-form cannot be predicted. *Emergent behaviour is always unpredictable* as it bears no direct relation to the individual properties of its component parts. The unpredictability of emergent behaviour does not fit well with science's emphasis on predictability!

In summary, if any new element is added to an existing system and the old and new elements combine, this creates a new and more complex system. This more complex system will exhibit its own new and unpredictable emergent behaviour.

In our previous examples of successful adaptation to a change of environment, the married couple and the traffic system managed to self-organise enough to maintain their form in a changing environment. The marriage survived the loss of the home. The traffic system kept going despite adverse weather conditions.

But when a new element is added at the level of the system itself, this represents a step up in complexity and 'emergent behaviour' is the consequence. If a new lover should tempt either husband or wife the outcome is unpredictable with potentially far reaching and ongoing consequences. The 'couple' has gone from two to three 'parts'. There may be a marriage break-up that will have knock-on effects, not just on the husband and wife but on their children and other relatives. The influence of the break-up can reverberate through generations.

In the same way, if a stray dog should venture onto the motorway it could disrupt the traffic system and cause an accident. This disastrous outcome can have unpredictable and far reaching consequences. The motorway traffic has gone from motor vehicles to motor vehicles and a stray dog. A part has been added to a system that was previously self-maintaining.

These consequences are all part of what is called emergent behaviour. Emergent behaviour, unpredictable as it may be, is a natural phenomenon.

Dimension 6 – the social dimension
The Family Unit, Friendship groups, School and Workforce, Sports teams, Societies, Populations (a chronological level with its own increasing complexity, both vertically and horizontally)

Dimension 5 – the organism
The Whole Person

Dimension 4 – different body systems and organs
The Brain and Central Nervous System

Dimension 3 – the multicellular dimension
Neuronal Circuits

Dimension 2 – the cellular dimension
Neurones

Dimension 1 – the biomolecular dimension
Hormones, Neurotransmitters, Enzymes

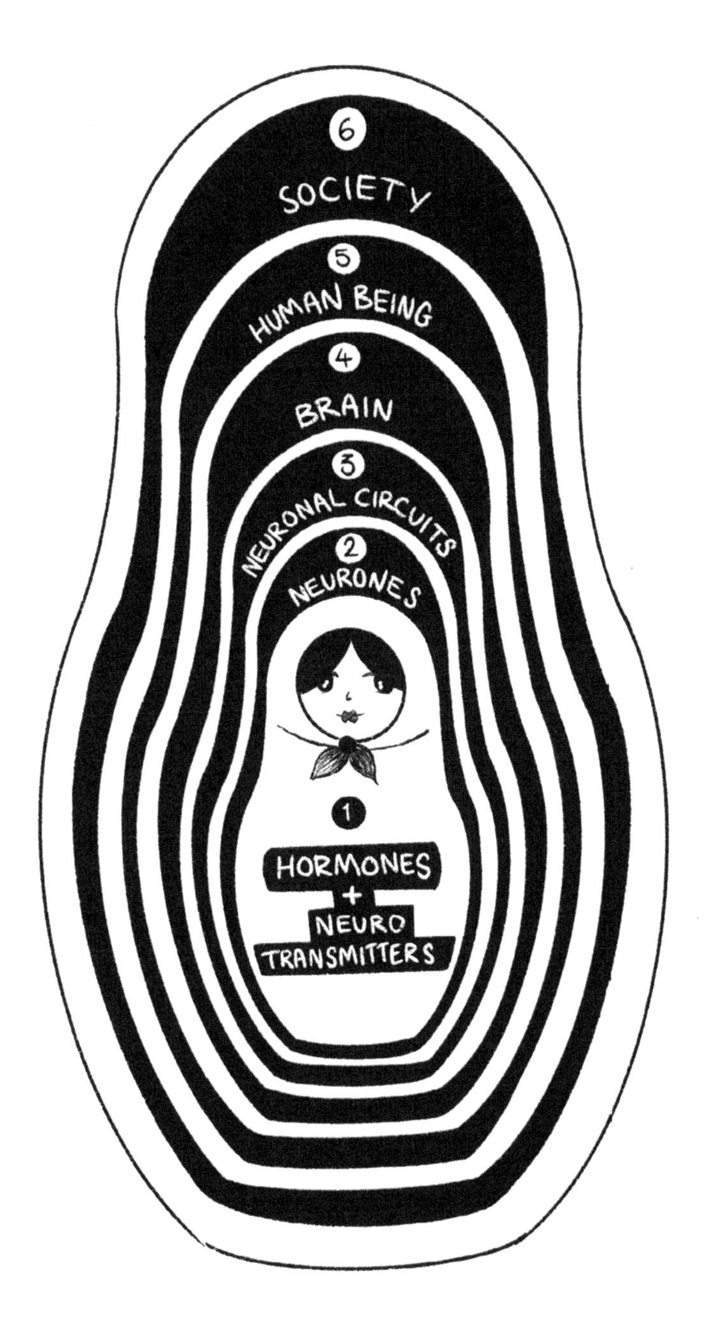

Figure 31. MENTAL HEALTH and the chronology of biological systems

'TOP DOWN' AND 'BOTTOM UP' EFFECTS

The ability of a system to self-organise and self-maintain is ultimately dependent on its environment. For the purpose of analysing behaviour, dependence of a system on its environment can be called a 'top down' effect.

The disruption caused by adding new parts to an established system, even if its environment is unchanged, will lead to emergent behaviour. This can be called a 'bottom up' effect.

All effects are a consequence of feed-back loops operating between the dimensions.

COMPLEXITY AND MENTAL HEALTH: THE DIMENSIONAL MODEL

A mental health patient can be considered as embodying a complex adaptive system. The different dimensions within that patient can be schematised as six dimensions, illustrated by the second Russian doll shown in figure 31. All the different dimensions will behave according to natural laws. Their individual behaviours will be influenced by their individual environments. If the environment is too challenging for the system at a particular dimension to remain as it is, the system will change its form. This is a 'top down' effect. If a new part is added to a system in one dimension there will be emergent behaviour, unpredictable in nature. This is a 'bottom up' effect on the whole complex adaptive biological system.

The 'lowest' of the biological dimensions is the biomolecular (D1).

TEN

THE BIOMOLECULAR DIMENSION (D1)

A COMPLEX SYSTEM

A biomolecule is a complex system where the atoms have a particular configuration and relationship in space. They self-organise as a consequence of the fields of force that exist between the atoms, and their ability to self-maintain is reliant on environmental conditions.

The basic biomolecular building blocks found in all organisms are lipids, amino acids, saccharides and nucleotides. These combine to form more complex biomolecules including the neurotransmitters essential for the transmission of information from one nerve cell to the next as well as hormones that circulate through the body; together these elements form the neuroendocrine system. Balance within this system is absolutely essential for the maintenance of psychological health. If the balance is tipped and there is an increased or decreased level of one neurotransmitter or hormone relative to another it can tip the patient into a completely altered mood or state of mind.

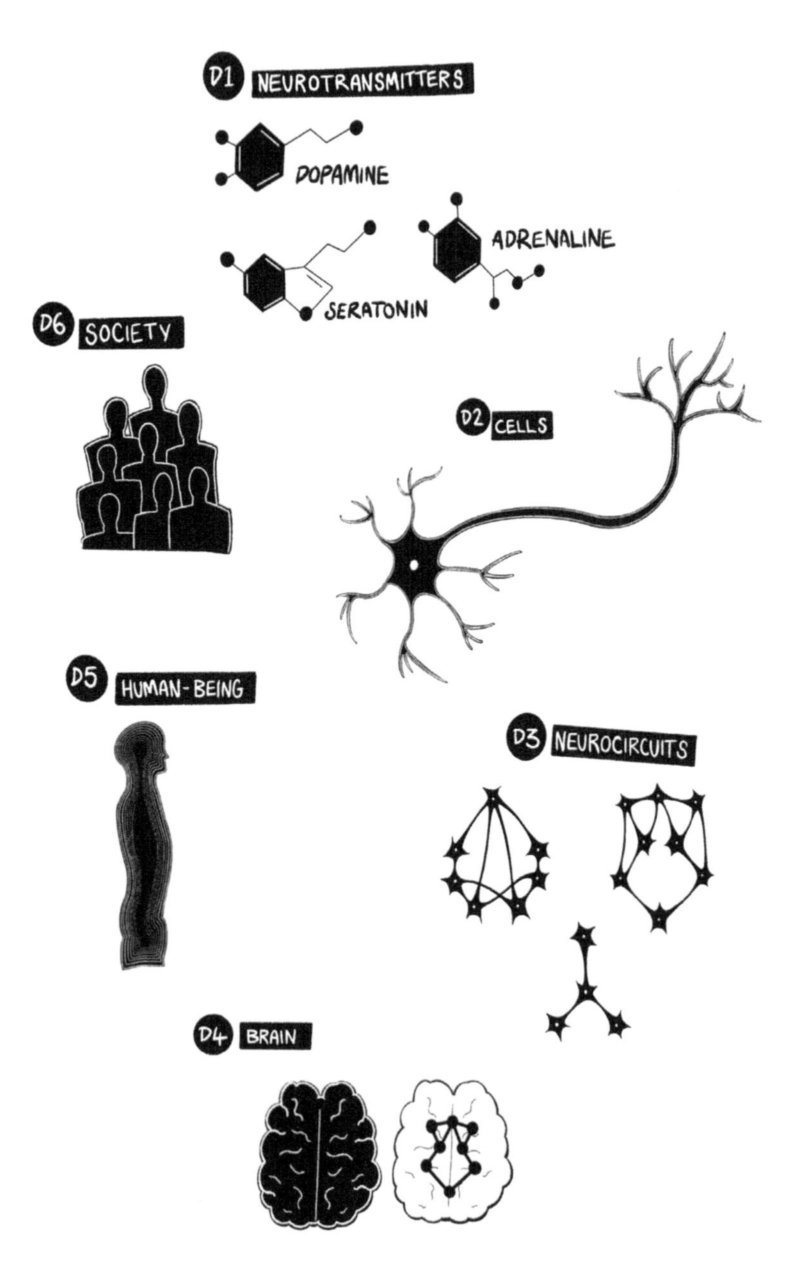

Figure 32. Biological complexity (dimensions D1–D6) in relation to mental health

DIAGNOSIS AT DIMENSION D1

The skill of a diagnostician lies in being able to understand whether the causative factor of a patient's suffering *originates* in the biomolecular dimension and, if so, which therapeutic approach that person should be directed towards. Heather, discussed below, is a patient who most likely struggles to hold her balance on two of Buser's spectrums (depression and anxiety – figures 22 and 24) as a consequence of a problem that originates at the biomolecular dimension.

Heather

Heather, a mother of four, grandmother of seven, has lived with a diagnosis of severe depression and anxiety since her mid-teens. Despite having suffered for near on 50 years, Heather is an extraordinary woman. Where one might imagine a sad, introverted and self-pitying soul, instead Heather is a loving, fun, supportive, generous beyond words and startlingly appealing woman.

But in her head, in her private world, she suffers. It is a constant battle managed with psychotropic drugs and self-help approaches that come and go endlessly, one after the other. At certain times, mainly at vulnerable hormonal stages of her life – puberty, post pregnancy and menopause – Heather's condition has spiralled into very severe episodes that even the drugs cannot control and where there is little anyone can do beyond keeping a very careful eye on her.

"I really believe" Heather told me with conviction, "that there *is* an answer out there somewhere that will release me from this medication." Although the drugs control her mood they also come with manifold side-effects, the most difficult to live with, day in and day out, she describes as "the flatness of everything". It is a sad fact that the drugs cannot always select which heightened emotions they dampen. Some of the more positive feelings that it would be good to hold onto get subdued along with the negative feelings, hence Heather's endless search for an alternative solution.

Heather is one of four children similarly affected by psychological issues and there is a long history on both the maternal and paternal sides, up and down through generations, of severe mental health problems, some of them psychotic in nature.

The relevance here is that the family history offers a chronology. Mental health issues are nothing new in this family. This could reflect learned behavioural patterns reaching back generations, but the cause is far more likely to be structural changes of biomolecular origin – probably something in the genes. The genes are the 'cookbooks' for the neurotransmitters and for the hormones. These need to be present in the correct quantity and quality for the brain to function well.

TREATMENT AT DIMENSION D1

If the metaphorical genetic cookbook has errors in the recipe this is a structural condition – 'a pathology' – that the body cannot reverse. In this situation no amount of altering the environment of the biomolecular soup will solve the problem. There has to be a direct intervention at the biomolecular level, most probably by the administering of psychotropic drugs – but only the right ones that will correct the errors without creating more. It is a delicate balancing act. Emergent behaviours will be a consequence, as parts are being added directly to the dimension that is to be influenced. These emergent behaviours include what are termed 'side-effects'. That is why they are so varied and unpredictable.

Maybe one day, with all the research now going into gene therapy and with increasing understanding of epigenetics (the study of how genes are switched on and off) some other form of treatment could develop. For the time being, assuming that the diagnosis of Heather's condition originating at the biomolecular dimension (D1) is correct and the drug is the best match available for the problem, Heather will need to keep putting up with the side-effect of the world around her seeming dulled. The alternative, to abandon the drug treatment, would only be worse.

Patients like Heather will need to see a doctor able to prescribe psychotropic drugs.

ELEVEN

THE CELLULAR DIMENSION (D2)

A COMPLEX ADAPTIVE SYSTEM

The next step up in complexity from the biomolecule is the cell – a dramatic leap up. This evolutionary step up was reliant on the presence of water and the interaction it has with the biomolecules. Water and specific biomolecules self-organise to form biological membranes.

The distinguishing feature of the cell, the unit of life, is the cell membrane: a structure that distinguishes intracellular from extracellular space by a continuous boundary. Cellular life depends on the cell boundary membrane for the exchange of matter, energy and information between the inside and the outside of the cell. Cells have life, in that they grow and multiply through a process of self-replication; to do this they extract energy from their environment. It is the advent of life that distinguishes a complex system from a complex *adaptive* system.

DIAGNOSIS AT THE LEVEL OF THE CELL (D2)

A patient whose suffering originates at the dimension of the cell (D2) can present with symptoms from any one or more of the eight spectrums of psychological health as described by Steven Buser (figures 22–29).

The dimension of the brain cell (the type of cell called a neurone) is rarely considered in the diagnosis of mental health problems. The neurones, of which there are many types, are composed of a cell body with axons and dendrons (nerve fibres) that receive and transmit impulses through electric discharges and the release of neurotransmitters (figure 32). The environment of these cells is the connective tissue or glial* cells.[68] When neurones start to become disorganised it is the surrounding environment that will need the attention of the therapist.

TREATMENT

At the nerve cell dimension (D2), the appropriate therapist would be one who can influence the general health of the connective tissue.

Health, for any bodily system from micro to macro, relies on the correct nutrients and oxygenation being available (uptake), a good circulatory system for delivery of these nutrients and removal of waste products locally (irrigation), and a healthy elimination system of the whole body (excretion). All three – uptake, irrigation and excretion – are required for a healthy connective tissue system that can support, connect and nourish the neurone.

Uptake

A nutritionist or medical herbalist can ensure that the correct nutrients to build the 'scaffolding' of the cell are being supplied, while a breathing expert can make sure that the correct balance of oxygen and carbon dioxide is entering the blood. Proper hydration is also extremely important.

* From the Greek word 'glia' meaning 'glue'.

Irrigation

In regard to the circulatory system, as well as efficient 'macro circulation' via the blood vessels and lymph system it is also important to have efficient 'micro-circulation', fluid movement in and out of cells – a significant aid to this being natural sunlight.[69]

Excretion

Finally, a good elimination system is vital to avoid the build-up of waste products in the connective tissue system. Good elimination is reliant on the health of the liver and the kidneys, and on an ability to sweat.

It may be that each of these systems needs supporting.

All of the above areas are addressed in the sometimes overwhelming volume of self-help advice that people are offered, but perhaps without any understanding of why or how each therapy contributes to the collective requirements of intake, irrigation and excretion. A good diet and regular breathing exercises will be far less beneficial if irrigation is poor or the elimination system is inadequate.

The connective tissue system of the brain forms the environment of the neurone, of the multi-neurone circuits and of the brain itself (respectively dimensions D2, D3 & D4). As a consequence, addressing the health of the connective tissue system through nutritional advice, self-help, supplements, exercise, fresh air, sunlight, good breathing and hands-on treatment will influence the environment of all three dimensions.

It should be noted here that addressing intake, irrigation and excretion in these ways will always benefit general health, but it will not significantly help a patient living with mental health problems when their condition originates in a *higher* dimension of biological complexity, namely the dimension of the individual (D5) or the social realm (D6).

TWELVE

THE MULTICELLULAR DIMENSION (D3)

Nerve cells (neurones) do not exist in isolation. They aggregate to become the networks and circuits comprising the multicellular dimension (D3). This is a dimensional level that can certainly be identified and targeted in patients (figure 32).[70] People develop problematic circuits in the brain within which small triggers can excite dramatic responses. When these responses are inappropriate and challenging for the patient personally and for those individuals close to them (as illustrated in the case study of Isaac below), the circuits need reorganising. How to approach this depends on where those circuits might be located in the brain.

Isaac

Isaac was ten months old when the authorities took him away from his parents. There had been reports of violence and Isaac had ended up in hospital. Isaac was adopted, finding a permanent loving home with a couple who, after having their first child, had discovered they were unable to conceive again. Isaac was nurtured, encouraged and above all loved, but as he entered his teens it became very apparent that Isaac was suffering psychologically. He became supersensitive – to noise in particular – and hyper-irritable.

At the point where I met the family everybody was tip-toeing around the house desperately trying to avoid anything that might trigger a reaction in Isaac. He would frequently fly into physical rages directed at members of the family or any physical objects in his path. Tables would be overturned, laptops thrown at windows; bruises and even fractures were inflicted by his flying fists and kicking feet. Once things calmed down Isaac displayed no sense of responsibility, only blaming those who had triggered him as the source of his irritation. That trigger could have been something as minor as a hiccup.

"And when he is calm," his parents added, "he becomes totally fixated, obsessive even, on inane subjects and we have to discuss them with him over and over again; it's as if the record is stuck and the stylus just can't escape from the groove."

Everyone hoped above hope that Isaac would emerge from what seemed to be a pubescent phase and this extreme behaviour would become a thing of the past. Time had moved on and so far that had not proved to be the case. He is 30 now and life has not been easy for him, his parents or his sibling.

Something happened to Isaac in the first ten months of his life, maybe even earlier. He was a victim of abuse, possibly more than once, which very likely triggered a fear response which in turn shaped a particular neuronal circuit in his unconscious mind or the 'primitive' area of the brain. The conscious part of his brain had not developed by ten months and for this reason no memory of the source of his fear is accessible to Isaac. He cannot remember what happened to lay down that particular brain circuitry at the very start of his life, yet the smallest trigger can stimulate it.

With that history, Isaac would possibly be diagnosed with PTSD. 'Normal' PTSD is commonly associated with soldiers coming back from the front line, torture victims, disaster survivors or children who have been subjected to physical, emotional or sexual abuse that they can remember. In these situations, the patient who can recall his or her trauma may have similar reactions to Isaac, but these will be linked to flashbacks drawing on a conscious memory. In Isaac's case there is no memory because of the timing of the trauma and so no flashbacks, only reactions. It is very likely that Isaac's problems originate at the multicellular level, in the form of inappropriate neuro-circuits located in the middle unconscious brain that are highly sensitised and fire off at the slightest stimulus.

Children who have suffered abuse from a young age commonly show an altered function of the *amygdala*, the two almond-sized areas of the brain located deep in the middle brain and representing our 'fear centres'.[71] The amygdala will likely be a very fundamental part of such inappropriate circuitry established during the very earliest stages of life. The amygdala relay messages of fear first to the body to stimulate a physiological response of 'fight or flight' to a frightening event (in Isaac's case this is often fight). At the same time they will relay, but at a slower speed, the sensation of fear to the conscious part of the brain where it can be registered.

DIAGNOSIS AT DIMENSION D3

A practitioner needs sufficient diagnostic skill to assess whether a patient is suffering at the multicellular level through inappropriate neuronal circuits which are either entirely subconscious, as in Isaac's case, or involve some conscious recognition by the patient of the events which caused the condition.

TREATMENT AT DIMENSION D3

Patients compromised at the multicellular level will, by virtue of their chronically traumatised state, almost inevitably have an imbalance too within the neuroendocrine system (D1), but this will represent a 'top down' effect, the source problem being at the 'higher' multicellular level (D3) impacting on the neuroendocrine balance in the biomolecular dimension below (D1). To treat such patients with drugs at the level of D1 may alleviate symptoms, but the target multicellular level (D3) that needs to be addressed to achieve a possible long-term solution will remain untreated. Treatment in such cases should be aimed directly at the multicellular level (D3) in an attempt to redirect the circuitry. There are specific practices that can target this level, tools that a qualified psychotherapist will have developed skills in, such as eye movement desensitization and reprocessing (EMDR), cognitive behavioural therapy (CBT) or maybe music and art therapies.

It was clear from Isaac's case history that he was struggling on the Personality spectrum that Buser describes (figure 29). The dimensional origin of the cause appeared to be the neuro-circuitry (D3). The fact that a trigger to this was probably from a very early age, of which he had no conscious memory, led me to recommend he find a psychotherapist with a specialist training in EMDR. I did not treat him.

Progress for Isaac has been slow but steady.

THIRTEEN

THE BRAIN (D4)

A COMPLEX ADAPTIVE SYSTEM

The next level of biological complexity is the dimension of 'systems and organs' (D4). Systems such as the central nervous system, the digestive system, the musculoskeletal system and the cardiovascular system and organs such as the heart, liver and – most importantly for mental health, the brain – arise from a combination of different multicellular tissue types.

BRAIN MAPPING

In the nineteenth century the orthodox medical profession began the process of what is termed 'brain mapping'. Scientists started to link specific functions (rather than emotions – this has come much later) to localised areas of the brain. The most famous loci to be discovered were 'Wernicke's area' for word recognition and 'Broca's area' for speech, both located in the left hemisphere.

Around the 1950s the emphasis of research changed. What is termed the 'mass action principle' postulated that brain function arose from a more complex action of all brain cells working together, rather than being localised. On this basis research moved rapidly away from specific physical localities of the brain towards understanding the biochemical processes of the whole brain. Existing treatments directed at the brain, such as the lobotomies and electroconvulsive therapy portrayed in the film *One Flew Over the Cuckoo's Nest*, rapidly declined in popularity. Subsequent treatment of mental health patients was no longer focused on the brain and its parts (D4) but shifted to the prescribing of psychotropic drugs which operate at the biomolecular dimension (D1). It all happened within a very short space of time.

Recently, diagnosis and treatment at the level of the brain, including treatment via its manipulation, is creeping back – albeit slowly. A new technology called 'functional brain imaging' is stimulating new interest among scientists who are discovering that certain locations in the brain are associated with specific emotions. This provides a new way of diagnosing by picking up visual changes in the brain.[72] This has led to research on potential treatment and the theory that activity at these particular loci can be manipulated by precisely placed electrodes or implanted 'pacemakers', although small progress has been made.[73]

DIAGNOSIS AT THE DIMENSION OF THE BRAIN (D4)

A patient suffering at the dimension of the brain (D4) can present with symptoms from any one or more of the eight spectrums of psychological health as described by Steven Buser.

The implants in the brain approach would represent a returning to diagnosis at this specific dimension. The treatment envisaged by the orthodox medical profession of placing a pacemaker or electrodes into the brain seeks to impose a change on specific parts of the brain implicated in a mental health problem. This is addressing the brain directly.

If the problem is only that the behaviour of that part of the brain has altered – there is no irreversible pathological change and the brain simply needs some help to change its behaviour –

then membrain disorder may be indicated. Before attempting to manipulate the brain itself it could be more appropriate to address the *environment* of that part of the brain, the relevant areas of the skull and dura which provide the housing and irrigation of the brain.

THE BRAIN'S ENVIRONMENT

This broader context – the *environment* of the brain – is never considered, as has been discussed in earlier parts of this book. The possibility that, in the case of a mental health issue, the brain could be struggling with a housing problem is seemingly absent from both the medical practitioner's and patient's mindset – and mindset is a difficult thing to change.

The skill of a practitioner here lies in being able to understand whether the origin of a patient's suffering is at the dimension of the brain (D4) and to what extent this suffering is a consequence of an abnormal environment (membrain disorder). Clues to this understanding can be found in the case history, observation and palpation of a patient.

PAST PATIENTS

At this point it is helpful to reintroduce Freddie, George, Amy, Dido and Eleanor whose stories were heard earlier. Each of these patients presented at my practice with psychological symptoms.

There may have been a number of factors contributing to the breakdown of their mental health in each case, but a causal factor common to all of these patients originated in the dimension of the brain (D4). Each had a problem with the *housing* of the brain, namely the skull, dura and irrigation system – that is to say, membrain disorder.

The existence of membrain disorder as a contributory factor at the dimension of the brain was discovered in each case by a combination of diagnostic techniques. These go beyond the normal range of diagnostic tools and skills available to medical and mental health practitioners for use with patients experiencing psychological problems. They include consideration of:

1. **The life-style of the patient** – especially any occupational or sports-related hazards
2. **Past medical history** – a general health overview, including *specifics* of accidents, operations, illnesses, and physical assaults. George had experienced two major head traumas as a child.
3. **Emotional health history** – periods of depression, anxiety, OCD etc.
4. **Past dental history** – Dido and Eleanor had both undergone orthodontic work, one as a child and the other as an adult.
5. **Visual observation** – Freddie had a significant plagiocephaly, Eleanor a less obvious asymmetry.
6. **Palpation** – in each patient the dura 'told a story' – in Amy's case it drew attention to a faint scar that might otherwise have gone unnoticed.

TREATMENT AT THE DIMENSION OF THE BRAIN (D4)

By this six-part investigation (which normally takes less than half an hour) it is possible to know whether or not the housing of the brain is abnormal. If it is, then the correct therapeutic intervention – a manual intervention – will normally help the patient significantly. The manual therapist would be trained in the cranial field and would use an indirect manual approach, perhaps over several treatments, to restore membrain health. The environment of the brain would be restored towards normal and, importantly, the irrigation system of the brain would improve. This will have an impact on the brain behaviour and consequent mood disorders and also an impact on the long-term health of the brain tissue.

It is also relevant to reintroduce the American footballer Aaron Hernandez (chapter 2). Well before the onset of the irreversible CTE brain disease discovered at autopsy, he was presenting with mood swings and problematic and sometimes violent behaviour. Aaron's lifestyle was typical of that of an American football player and, as such, he certainly suffered repetitive head injuries from high school onwards and probably before.

Professional sports teams have a whole array of support staff to keep their players at the top of their game both psychologically and physically. It is suggested that they should also have a manual therapist trained in the cranial field who would assess players regularly, always at the end of each season and especially after any impacts to the head.

Once there is a pathological change to the brain tissue itself, this is irreversible and a referral to a neurologist is appropriate.

FOURTEEN

THE WHOLE PERSON (D5)

A COMPLEX ADAPTIVE SYSTEM

The next level up in complexity is the whole person. A human being is a complex adaptive system which self-forms through the embryological and growth process and self-maintains, constantly adapting its behaviour according to environmental conditions.

MENTAL HEALTH

When looking at the dimension of the individual or whole person (D5), it is a widely accepted view that a person's environment influences their mental state. There has been a rapid increase in scientific and medical awareness of how nature, fresh air, sunlight and exercise have extraordinarily beneficial effects on a person's mental health.

What can be described as the 'environment' of an individual means far more than whether their time is spent in a city or the countryside, outside in the fresh air or cooped up in a small flat. Human beings are social beings and 'environment' covers a very broad range of possible influential elements – friends and family, home and work situation, health, financial situation, traumatic events. These conditions may be ongoing or part of someone's past. An environmental influence on an individual's mental state might be as simple as encountering a new challenge in life with the stress of adapting to new and different circumstances. The impact of a sudden change in environmental circumstances on an individual (D5) is illustrated in the story of Peter.

Peter

Peter and his siblings, parents and grandparents have been patients of mine, seeing them intermittently, over decades. His mother originally brought Peter for a consultation some months after a car accident when he was two years of age. He received a head injury that directly damaged the left side of his brain. At that age the brain has a plasticity that makes the outcome of such an injury unpredictable. Undamaged areas of the brain take over the roles of those areas that are damaged. My osteopathic attention was directed only towards the skull and underlying membrane system that had also been subjected to the trauma. My treatment, I hope, had the effect of providing the best possible environment for the injured brain.

It was evident by the time Peter was a teenager that the legacy of the brain injury was a mild speech problem and an element of clumsiness. Otherwise he had no other symptoms, he thrived at school and was clever and funny. He avoided sports and much preferred one-to-one conversations rather than having to compete in a big group. Peter was one of four and the family was a happy one.

Peter thrived until he left his supportive home and went off to university, found himself in halls surrounded by large groups of confident and articulate students and became conscious of the difficulty that he had engaging in group conversations. Unusually for him, he felt fretful and underconfident. He was excelling in his studies, but it wasn't enough to lift his spirits and he decided to look for help by going to the campus GP surgery.

The GP sent him into the waiting room to fill in a multiple-choice questionnaire, the PHQ-9 depression test.[74] The answers to nine questions are added up to give a diagnostic score and Peter's score indicated 'social anxiety'. The GP wanted to send Peter for some counselling but the waiting list was long. Instead, he offered him a prescription of a well-known antidepressant of the 'serotonin reuptake inhibitor' class (probably the best known of these in the UK is Prozac).

The kind of medication that Peter was prescribed has a long list of possible side-effects, the most severe of which is suicidal impulses.[75,76,77] The particularly dangerous times are at the beginning of taking the medication and after the patient has come off it. Peter took the drug for six weeks and then, thinking that he was fine again, started to come off the medication. He had settled into university, had found a cohesive group of friends and his confidence was building again. He was adapting to his new environment over time.

It was in that first week of cutting down on the medication that Peter tragically died by suicide. It is impossible even to begin to describe the shock and the grief for all concerned.

Peter's story is not an uncommon one.

Some patients who seek the help of their GP or psychiatrist will have had severe, debilitating, long-standing anxiety or depression which has stopped their life in its tracks, perhaps over years. They might have been unable to work or take care of their children, their mental pain so intense that each day felt like a form of crucifixion. It may be that other treatments had not worked. In such cases, this kind of drug offers a possible solution and might be worth a try, despite its alarming side-effects.

That makes some sense. Peter's case made no sense.

Peter had no history of mental health problems before approaching his GP. A list of symptoms ticked on a multiple choice form and checked against the DMS manual was enough to satisfy a diagnostic label and trigger the prescription of a potentially lethal drug.

It might be assumed that Peter suffered with depression simply because of an old brain injury, but this would be to ignore the timing of his depression and the environmental change that triggered it. He had since infancy lived with a very mild disability affecting his speech and dexterity or coordination such that, when he arrived at university, surrounded by confident-sounding students, he stood apart from the cool crowd. His mild disability had had little to no impact when his environment was familiar, it simply made it more difficult for him to adapt to a new environment.

Peter had left his warm loving family, home, friends and the territory he had been familiar with throughout his life. Many students experience the same kind of difficulty to a greater or lesser degree. In Peter's case he did not die by suicide because he was having problems adapting to a new setting, but because of a known potential side-effect of a psychotropic drug. This drug influenced Peter at the biomolecular dimension (D1), which was not the dimension of origin of his mental health issue. The drug did nothing to resolve the problem originating at the dimension of the individual (D5) – adapting to a changed social environment. Instead, it turned a difficulty into a tragedy.

This is a very sad story and is told only to illustrate the dangers of not addressing the correct dimension of origin at which a patient might be struggling. Peter didn't need drugs. He didn't have membrain disorder. He didn't need EMDR or CBT. The story of Peter provides a graphic illustration of how treating a patient at the wrong diagnostic dimension on the basis of a DMS label can have unnecessary and catastrophic consequences. Peter was treated as if he had a problem at the biomolecular level (D1) when in fact it was the whole person (D5) in relation to his new environment that was suffering. Peter needed talking therapy.

The GP was reprimanded for prescribing the medication without ensuring that there was an adult over 21 who could closely supervise Peter whilst he was on the drug. It had not been the GPs first choice of treatment – this was talking therapy, however local funding had not made this accessible. This, of course, is a different conversation. Suffice to say that if the correct cause of an illness could be identified and matched with the correct treatment right at the start, not only could devastating incidents such as Peter's suicide be prevented, but the amount of money that the NHS would save would be huge.

DIAGNOSIS AND TREATMENT AT THE DIMENSION OF THE WHOLE PERSON (D5)

A patient suffering at the dimension of the whole person (D5) can present with symptoms from any one or more of the eight spectrums of psychological health as described by Steven Buser. A patient, at the time of presenting to a practitioner and asking for help, will have shifted to an extreme spectral range where normal life becomes out of reach. They may be anxious, suffering with OCD, paranoia, attention deficit or a combination of these and more. As a practitioner, having recognised on which spectrum or spectrums a patient is suffering, the next thing to consider is in what dimension is the *cause* of the suffering, so that it can be successfully addressed.

Diagnosis at the level of D5 will become apparent by talking to the patient and (at its most simplistic!) understanding what is going on in their life and what has gone on in the past. In many cases it will be obvious. There may be the death of a loved one, divorce, family trauma, bullying at work – the list is endless. If the *cause* of the imbalance on the spectrum is at the level of the whole person then the environment of the individual needs to be addressed and this is where talking therapy is the best approach. A talking therapist will help the patient to understand what it is in their environment, whether past or present, that is causing their imbalance. Through this understanding the patient has the potential to move away, change or adapt around the environmental stress or stresses.

If the *cause* of a patient's suffering is at the dimension of the individual (D5) it can have an impact on the circuitry in their brain (D3). These patients may well go over and over a situation in their heads. The neuroendocrine system (D1) too will be affected by raised levels of certain chemicals in the brain and in the bloodstream. The cranial membranes may react as they do in situations of fear and stress by becoming long and narrow (D4) (figure 5). These are all 'top down' effects. If these patients are treated with psychotropic drugs or some sort of manual therapy aimed at releasing tension, it may well help them, but these approaches are not addressing the *cause*. They need talking therapy.

FIFTEEN

SOCIETIES (D6)

A COMPLEX ADAPTIVE SYSTEM

Human beings are social beings and, as individuals, rarely exist in isolation. They tend to share their lives and it is these groups of people that make up the next layer of complex adaptive systems – collectively termed here as societies (D6).

There are many different relationships that each individual plays a part in and these relationships occupy many different levels of complexity, extending both vertically and horizontally.

An individual may have a partner, children and parents. This immediate family will branch out into an extended family, a step-family, in-laws, and so on. This same individual may be part of a work force, a sports team, a group of old university or school friends or a religious group, perhaps. The same person is a member of a local geographical community, itself part of a larger population, regional, national or even global.

Societies, despite their differences, follow the same natural laws as any other complex adaptive system. Groups of people or societies, however small or however big, self-organise and self-maintain, adapting constantly to changes in their environment by changing their behaviour. If those environmental changes become too stressful and the group or society is unable to maintain its form it may, as history shows, break apart into smaller societies and/or join forces with other groups in order to become more robust.

At the time of writing this book the global population is into the third year of the Covid-19 pandemic, the climate crisis appears to be accelerating at an alarming rate and there is mass migration in different parts of the world as a consequence of conflicts, climate change and social and economic instability and inequality.

There are broadly speaking two options available to individual governments and regional alliances in the face of these threatening challenges of the global environment. One is to seek collective global action, every country joining forces and developing a collegiate approach on the basis that global problems have no respect for political borders and will inevitably affect us all. The other choice is for individual countries to close geographical boundaries and hunker down; a smaller complex system is typically more adaptable and agile than a cumbersome, giant and highly complex system and while not all smaller systems would survive, some might.

This is an example of the polarisation seen whenever systems are under extreme stress and unable to self-maintain their present form. A polarised system is intrinsically unstable and its outcome unpredictable. In this context, it is unsurprising that mental health issues abound even in societies which have for decades enjoyed relative peace and stability.

MENTAL HEALTH AT THE LEVEL OF GROUPS AND SOCIETIES (D6)

A group of people suffering at the societal dimension (D6) can present with collective and varied symptoms along any one or more of the eight spectrums of psychological health described by Steven Buser.

On the smaller scale it may be that the inhabitants of a village, town or whole country are affected mentally by having to live through natural disasters such as war, flooding or fires. There may be a segment of a population who have had to flee their countries and are homeless – as seen in the ever-rising refugee crisis. Minority ethnic and religious groups routinely suffer bullying and discrimination within their own country. The poor are typically exploited by the rich.

The difference between the dimension of society (D6) and that of the individual (D5) is that in the case of a social group, the causative factors of at least some pressing mental health problems are 'built in' to that entire group's life experience. Increasingly, with the growth of global communications and global economic interdependency, the social group is the global population.

DIAGNOSIS AND TREATMENT

Diagnosing and treating mental health issues originating at the social level (D6) is an enormous subject that goes well beyond the scope of this book. Addressing the *causes* of mental health issues at the social level requires first of all that politicians, businesses, media and technology giants, social movements and other influential bodies and individuals take mental health at least as seriously as physical health, and work with the same resolve as is shown in the arena of physical health to remedy psychological problems which can be made better or made worse by their decisions and actions.

Solving society's problems does not help people living with mental health issues if the causes of their suffering have a biological origin – from the dimensions of D1–D4.

Those whose decisions can affect the mental health of individuals, groups and societies should therefore be aware that mental health issues also have biological origins, not all of which have received sufficient research attention. One example is membrain disorder, discussed in detail in Part One of this book.

SIXTEEN

A MULTI-DIMENSIONAL DIAGNOSIS

Up to this point the impression may have been given that a mental health problem originates in just one biological or social dimension, but this is not always the case. In many patients there may be multiple causative factors stemming from different dimensions. If the different dimensions can be identified, then a coordinated treatment approach can be orchestrated.

Jack

Jack was 23 when he walked into my practice. As with so many of the young adult patients who find their way to me, it was his parents who had taken charge and arranged the appointment. Jack had left a good job in journalism (his passion), unable to cope with the daily demands of a full-time job and sharing a flat with his friends. He had moved back home. "He's been struggling with depression now for the last ten years or so, but we've never seen him like this," said his mother. "He has no enthusiasm to do anything for himself, not even to read a book, see a friend, go for a walk. He seems completely incapacitated and we just don't know how to help him." Jack's world was getting darker, more lonely and sadder by the day.

Jack had been seeing psychiatrists since he was fifteen years old. He had been given almost as many different labels for his condition as years he had been under the mental health care team. Jack himself filled me in. "They've told me I have irritable depression combined with social anxiety disorder." The latter is summarised in DSM-5 as an intense, persistent fear of being watched and judged by others. Depression is summarised as experiencing symptoms of sadness, loss of interest, guilt, energy loss, concentration loss, appetite change, psychomotor changes, sleep change and suicidal thoughts for more than two weeks.

Jack was on a cocktail of medications and they were not working. At the stage of his initial consultation with me he was taking four different medications for his mental health. There had been no solution found in eight years; in fact Jack was in a worse state than he had ever been.

I took Jack's case history and examined him both visually and through palpation.

JACK'S CASE HISTORY

Jack had grown up in a household with a very anxious and depressed mother. There was mental illness on both sides of the extended family and up through the previous generations. Jack had received orthodontic treatment during two periods of his life, the first around 13 years old and then again around 21 years old. He was about 22 when his mental health, always bad, had rapidly deteriorated. He began to suffer uncontrollable panic attacks which meant that he could not leave the house.

Jack suffered from what he himself described as a poor immune system, with repeated episodes of acute tonsilitis forcing him to take lengthy doses of strong antibiotics at least two or three times a year. He suffered with acne and the development of cysts in different areas of his body.

OBSERVING JACK

Jack was hunched, his body assuming the characteristic posture of someone who is depressed or anxious. His skin was pale and covered with acne. There was a visible plagiocephaly that reflected in the asymmetry of his nose and a jaw that deviated strongly to the left side.

On close observation it was possible to see that the tonsils were chronically enlarged and reddened, suggesting a low-grade chronic inflammation.

PALPATING JACK

The conflict between cranial base, jaw and middle face was evident in the reactivity and pull of the membrane system when I palpated Jack's skull. This conflict was not restricted to the cranium but reflected through the entire body. When a patient is in a state of

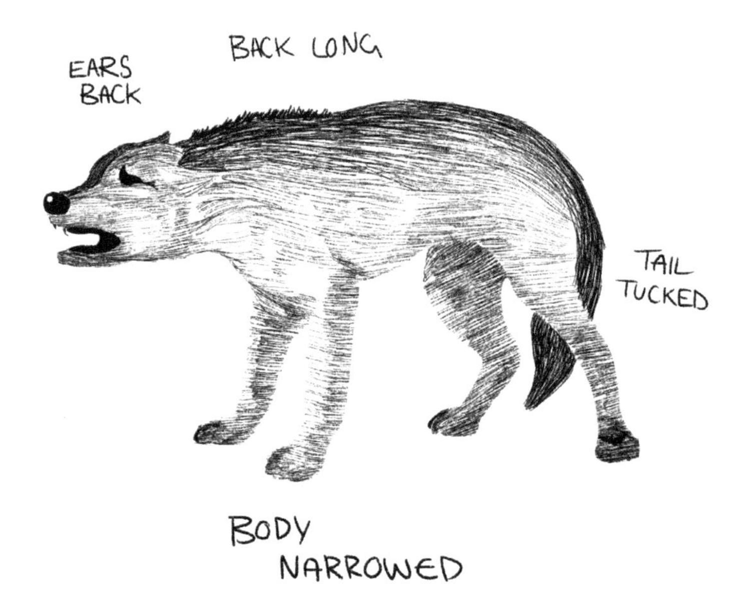

Figure 33. A physical manifestation of anxiety visible in a dog reflects the same but invisible response of the dural membrane system in the dura.

extreme anxiety their entire membrane system will respond in such a way that the whole dura 'tadpole' system, the central axis of the entire fascial system, will become narrow and elongated and lock into that state (see figure 5, C).

It is a physical manifestation of a state of high arousal: in this case extreme alertness combined with fear.

This physical response is visible outwardly on a dog. When a dog is about to fight, or flee, the ears will flatten backwards as the spine and back lengthens (figure 33). The frightened dog offers a visible representation of what happens to the dura, invisible within a human being, in a similar situation. The dura is, however, palpable. That was Jack. The membrane system pulling up, up and further up, physically maintaining a state of high arousal that Jack could not possibly release by himself. This is classic in patients who suffer panic attacks.

DIAGNOSIS AND APPROPRIATE TREATMENTS

My diagnosis of Jack indicated that Jack needed treatments to address causative factors in a combination of different dimensions.

The fact that there was a history of depression and anxiety within Jack's direct household raised the possibility of learned behaviour. Recent research has shown that a new type of psychological intervention between children and the anxious parent at an early stage in the child's life can have some success in breaking this generational hand-me-down. The *Let's talk about the children* programme offers an e-learning resource to parents with mental health problems.[78] Unfortunately, if this would have helped Jack as a child, it was too late for him as an adult to embark on such a programme.

It was also possible, given that there were mental health issues running through both the paternal and maternal lines, that there was a genetic basis to his condition. This would require the intervention of a psychiatrist and the administration of the correct medication for a disorder at the biomolecular dimension (D1). However, treatment at this level alone would not be sufficient.

The condition of Jack's skin was relevant. Acne is a sign of excessive cyst formation and cyst formation signals a failure of the body to eliminate waste. The cysts lock the waste products into a sphere rather than eliminating them to the outside surface and the sphere remains in the body. The same is true of the tonsils which trap the very infection that the system is trying to be rid of. Both tonsillitis and acne are signs of a toxic connective tissue environment. This is the very same connective tissue that includes the dura which houses, supports and nourishes our brain.

The cause of the body's failure to eliminate waste effectively is most likely to be a combination of inappropriate intake (in whatever form) and a failing elimination system. Toxic drugs are broken down primarily in the liver and medication can put an extreme stress on the liver and also the kidneys. A stressed liver creates a poor metabolic environment, incapable of dealing properly with the waste products.

Remember that Jack's intake included a cocktail of four psychotropic drugs and regular long doses of strong antibiotics. Jack needed advice on how to support his liver.

As for Jack's tonsils, regular doses of antibiotics were clearly not the long-term solution to his problem. The tonsils, harbouring a persistent source of infection, repeatedly challenged his immune system and probably restricted good air flow from the nose through to the lungs. The tonsils needed to come out.

Jack also needed a manual therapist trained in the cranial field. The dura, the bag that the brain sits in, desperately needed some hands-on help. The dura first needed to be released from its elongated and narrow state so that the feedback loop of panic feeding his high levels of anxiety could be broken. The next part of a manual therapy approach would be to try to support the self-correcting dura to deal with the conflict around the jaw and middle face which the dura was – amongst other things – trying to resolve.

The information that I gathered from Jack by taking his case history and observing and palpating him told me that there were multi-system dimensions implicated here and he required appropriate help at each of those levels. Jack's mental health issues had to be addressed at different levels and a multi-therapist approach needed to be orchestrated – one with a clear rationale. Jack did indeed need a psychiatrist, because the genetic inheritance issue (D1) could only be addressed with the right drugs. He also needed a surgeon to remove the tonsils and a nutritional therapist (a medical herbalist, nutritionist or naturopath) who would work appropriately to support the liver; both interventions would aim to improve the connective tissue environment (D2, D3 and D4). Jack needed a manual therapist trained in the cranial field to resolve the tensions and distortions of the dura and cranium and restore normal housing to the brain as far as possible – to re-establish membrain health (D4).

So, what happened?

TREATMENT AND OUTCOME

I treated Jack seven times and his mental health started to improve, gradually but significantly. Treatment was aimed first at releasing the dura from its long narrow state which had been locking him into a vicious cycle of anxiety. The next stage was to try to support the dura to reconcile the conflict between jaw, middle face and the cranial base.

By the fourth treatment Jack was starting to develop an interest in himself. He started reading books and going out for short runs. Around treatment five I encouraged Jack to have his tonsils out as I believed them to be a constant aggravating factor that would prevent a stable recovery. Jack told me that he was keen for this, but the doctors told him they did not think that such an intervention was warranted.

Jack wanted to start going out and socialising again but was worried about his acne. Jack was advised by his doctor to start yet another medication, along with his other psychotropic drugs, in this case further antibiotics for six to eight weeks to "cure the acne". I advised against it. I talked to the parents, I talked to Jack, but the decision to go ahead and take the drugs was made, between them and the GP.

I honestly felt that I had a better understanding of Jack and his psychological and physical illness and how they could be appropriately treated than the psychiatrists who had been seeing Jack for more than eight years. Treatment via the dura had brought about significant improvements. I understood a lot of the factors contributing towards his chronically poor mental health which, up to the point of consulting me, had proved untreatable and was deteriorating. The psychiatrist, the parents, and Jack himself were unaware of these contributory factors. I tried to explain them to the parents but it was decided at that point that the GP and psychiatrist knew best and that was the last I saw of Jack.

Prior to the prescription of further acne drugs, Jack had made a point of thanking me effusively for the difference that my osteopathic approach had made. I had always known that my manual therapy would not be enough to hold the correction without bringing other colleagues alongside to complement what I was doing in the dimension of the brain. I didn't have time or indeed the power to orchestrate that team approach for Jack's benefit before a yet further assault was inflicted on his metabolism by the introduction of the acne drug.

A VISUALISATION OF JACK

Figure 34 is a visualisation of the difference between normal housing of the brain and the abnormal housing of Jack's brain, based on

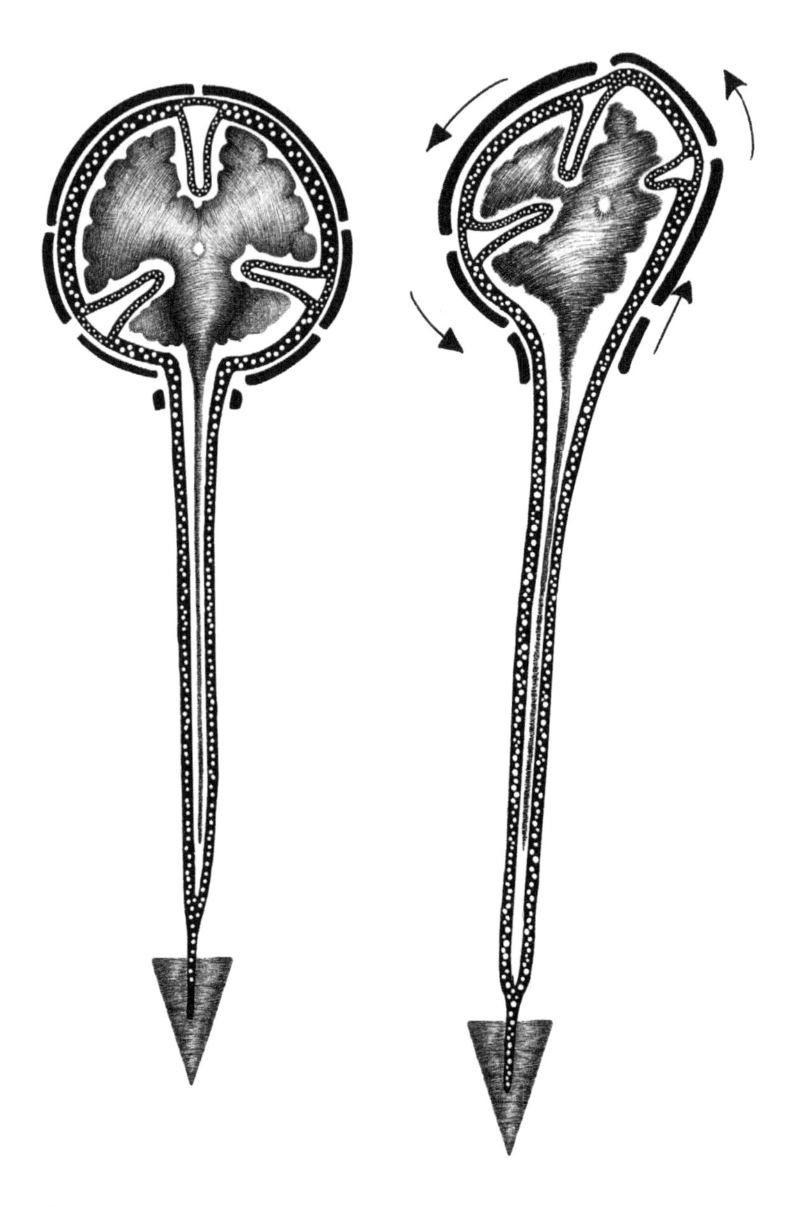

Figure 34. A visualisation comparing 'normal' housing of the brain (left) and Jack's membrain disorder (right).

observing and palpating his cranium. In Jack, all compartments of the skull were distorted, including the upper compartments which house the frontal and parietal lobes, part of our cerebral cortex (linked to consciousness).

The picture also shows (right) an anti-clockwise torsion or twisting through the central compartment of the brain. This area houses the midbrain or unconscious part of the brain.

Understanding which parts of the brain are associated with which emotions and where these parts of the brain sit within the skull offers clues as to whether these areas might be influenced by membrain disorder in the form of decreased space, distortion, compression or congestion – or, most likely, a combination of these.

SEVENTEEN

REGIONS OF THE BRAIN

The regions of the brain are often described in terms of the brain's different stages of evolutionary development.[79]

THE 'PRIMITIVE' OR 'HIND' BRAIN

The *hind brain* is the oldest part of the brain in evolutionary terms. It is located deep in the floor of the *cranial fossa* (cavity), near the back. It sits above the densely formed cranial base and is thus heavily protected (figure 35). This is no accident. It is natural selection at work, favouring the most secure housing of the vital control centres for life. The hind brain is concerned with body regulation: respiratory rate, heart rate, temperature control, blood pressure and other vital mechanisms. Without this regulation death is instant. The *cerebellum* (Latin for 'the small brain') is part of the hind brain and is responsible for orientation and movement. While the floor of the hind brain is the hard cranial base, its roof comprises the horizontal dividers of the pliable dural membrane system (see figure 37).

Irrigation of this area is via the arteries that wind around the top of the *cervical spine* bringing blood to the area and a complex

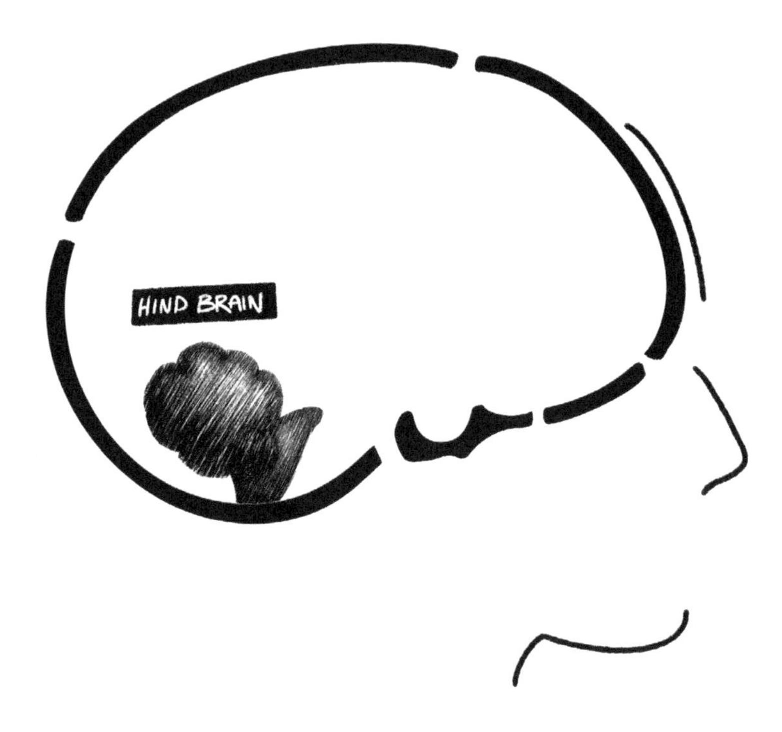

Figure 35. Hind brain

network of tiny veins (the *venous plexus*) through which the blood passes back out of the cranium. The hind brain nestles upon this plexus, almost as on a pillow.

THE MIDDLE BRAIN

Forward of and slightly above the hind brain is the middle brain or *midbrain* (figure 36). The midbrain has an array of locations associated with different functions. These include the *thalamus* – a relay centre, directing information to all the different parts of the brain like an old-fashioned telephone exchange, the *hypothalamus* and *pituitary gland* – a collection of condensed areas that manage the homeostatic regulation of our body through our hormones and nervous systems, the *hippocampus* and amygdala which are

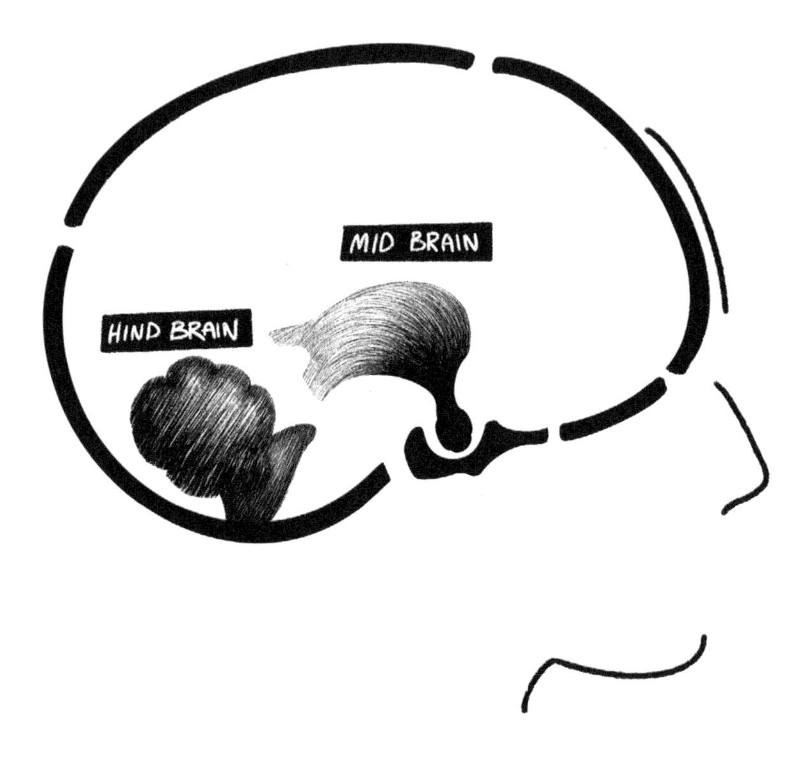

Figure 36. The midbrain

the centres for long-term and emotional memories, and the *limbic system* – the emotional centres. The midbrain is responsible for the basic instincts that help to keep us alive, healthy, and able to procreate – our survival instincts.

While the middle brain or midbrain sits slightly above and forward of the hind brain, it too is seated on the floor of the sturdy cranial base. It is surrounded by the edges of the horizontal and vertical dividers of the dura in a space that is unlikely to become compressed as it is exceptionally well protected (figure 37). However if the dura is sufficiently distorted then this space can become distorted with it (figure 34).

The midbrain sits on what is called the 'circle of Willis', an arterial roundabout where blood entering into the skull circulates

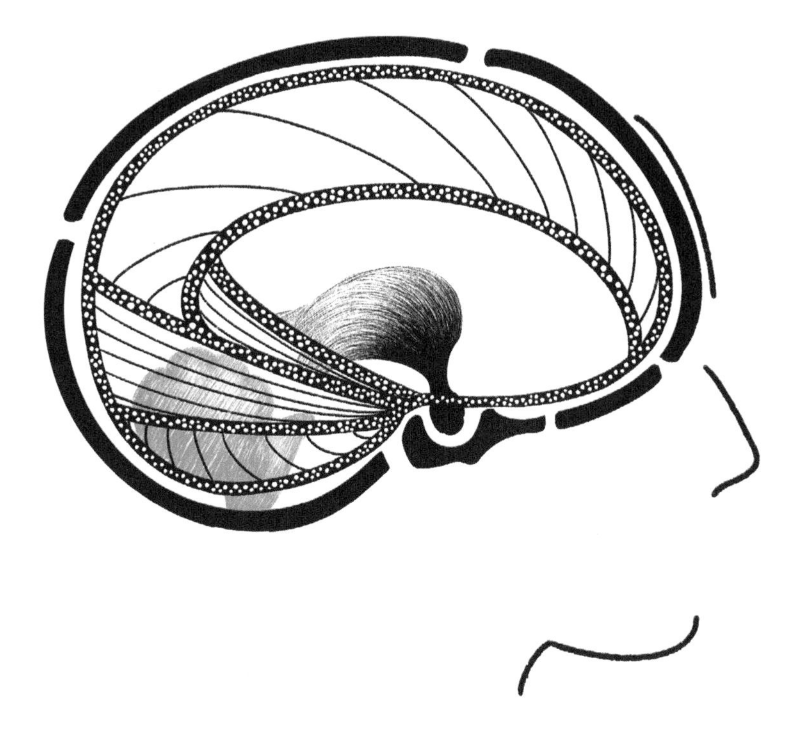

Figure 37. The hind brain sits on the sturdy cranial base and is roofed by the dura's horizontal dividers. The midbrain sits on the cranial base and is surrounded above and to each side by edges of both vertical and horizontal dividers.

before being diverted out to the more peripheral parts of the brain. The edges of the vertical and horizontal dividers of the dura contain the venous sinuses, blood vessels that propel the blood back, downwards and out of the skull. Exactly as with a traffic system, if there are any bottlenecks or blockages on any one of the highways, particularly the exits from the highways (the veins), then congestion and diversion of fluids from their proper course is the outcome. A distortion in the dura can have these effects.

The middle and hind brain are both unconscious. In *The Chimp Paradox* by psychiatrist Steve Peters, the unconscious brain is referred to as 'the chimp'. It is emotional, reactive, irrational, visceral, sensitive, playful, childish, but at the same time essential for our survival. It is present in every one of us.[80]

THE CEREBRAL HEMISPHERES

The cerebral hemispheres were the next part of the brain to evolve as part of the expansion of the brain (which occurred in the relatively short evolutionary time period between 800,000 and 200,000 years ago). This part of the brain channels our conscious thoughts. It is divided into various lobes which exist in pairs, left and right (figure 38).

The *occipital lobes* are at the back and form the visual processing area.

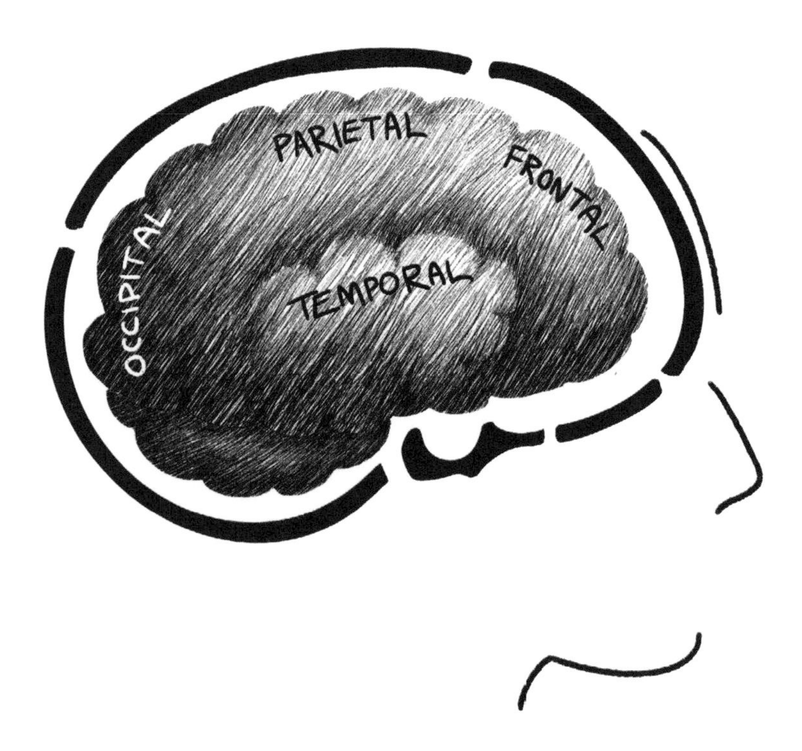

Figure 38. Cerebral hemispheres

The *parietal lobes* sit atop the brain and are mainly concerned with sensation and movement.

The *temporal lobes* are situated on either side of the brain. The left temporal lobe holds the faculty of speech and word recognition and both lobes hold some aspects of memory.

Finally, the frontal lobes, unsurprisingly, are found at the front. The frontal lobes are what make us distinctively human. Their development has led to what we call 'consciousness'. They allow for such fundamental human features as a sense of self, a sense of purpose, an ability to concentrate and organise the mind and, importantly, to reflect on ourselves and control our instinctual urges so that we do not disgrace ourselves socially or behave criminally – for the most part. This part of the brain Professor Peters refers to as 'the human'. It, like 'the chimp', is present in every one of us and it marks us as human.

The whole cerebral cortex comprising these elements is roofed, walled and floored by a combination of the cranial vault and the vertical and horizontal dividers of the dura, which create compartments. There is a malleability associated with these structures, composed as they are of membrane and thin bony plates that fit together like a three-dimensional jigsaw puzzle. It is because the housing has a degree of malleability that distortion is possible.

The frontal lobes have been studied extensively and in certain behavioural or emotional conditions different parts of the lobes have been shown to be underactive or overactive.[81] Figure 39 shows which areas of the frontal lobes are considered to be associated with which mental states.

FRONTAL LOBE HOUSING

As a generalisation, areas around the midline of the frontal lobe influence a person's inner experience of themselves while the more peripheral areas are concerned with a person's relationship with the

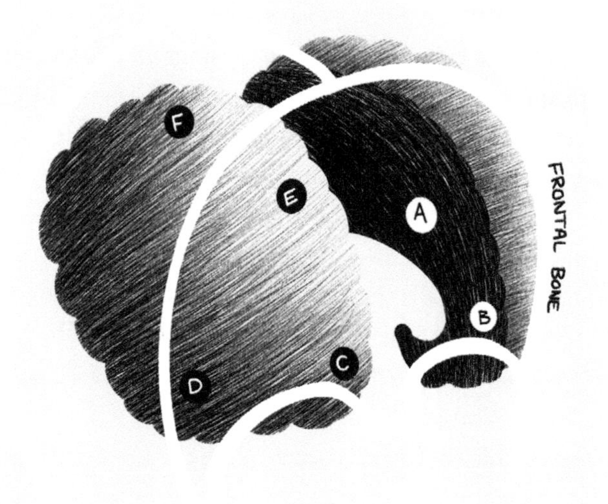

- A FOCUSED ATTENTION (↑ ACTIVITY OCD + DEPRESSION)
- B EMOTIONS EXPERIENCED (↑ ACTIVITY DEPRESSION)
- C INHIBITION OF URGES (↓ ACTIVITY INAPPROPRIATE BEHAVIOUR)
- D EMPATHY (↓ ACTIVITY ASPERGERS + SOCIOPATHS)
- E GENERATING PLANS + BUILDING CONCEPTS (↓ ACTIVITY IN DEPRESSION)
- F WHOLE BODY IMAGE IN RELATION TO OUTER WORLD (↓ ACTIVITY IN WITHDRAWAL)

Figure 39. Different locations of the right and left hemispheres associated with different emotions. Their positions are shown relative to their bony housing.

outer world. If a patient is living with mental health issues, one of the possibilities to consider is whether the altered behaviour of the frontal lobes might be associated with a disorder in their housing; namely that the patient is suffering with membrain disorder.

The frontal lobes fit snugly into the caved shape of the frontal bone (figure 39). This cave-shaped cavity is divided into left and right compartments by the vertical divider of the dura. This divider sits in continuity with the vertical divider of the nose and nasal cavity. Patients tend not to attach much significance to a broken nose, a cosmetic nose operation or a procedure to open up the sinuses, yet each of these represents a trauma to the middle face which will have consequences for whatever exists in continuity above – namely the vertical divider of the dura.

If the midline divider is distorted or compressed it may well, because of its proximity to the middle part of the frontal lobe, influence the way a patient feels 'in' themselves. For example, a patient may complain of poor attention and an inability to focus for any length of time. They may become fixed on a thought that they cannot let go of – in other words, the patient is depressed. The story, in the Author's Foreword to this book, of my own broken nose and the operation to repair it, illustrates how this might happen.

Alternatively, a blow to the forehead, to the crown of the head, to the area around the eye or to the side of the head has the potential to impair the relationship of the frontal bone with its many neighbours, affecting the housing of the frontal lobes and potentially influencing the individual's whole body image in relation to the outer world. A patient suffering in this way may come in complaining of a sense of disconnectedness and an inability to form relationships with people.

On the outer aspect of the right frontal lobe there is an area associated with empathy (labelled D in figure 39). This area is linked with the ability to 'put oneself into another's shoes' –

something absent to a greater or lesser extent in those diagnosed with autism or in sociopathy.[82,83,84] Those with autism do seem to benefit from osteopathic intervention. Sociopaths however are famous for lacking any acknowledgment of their own condition and so are extremely unlikely to seek treatment.

Osteopathic colleagues have many parents who bring their autistic children in the hope that osteopathy can help, but with little to no understanding of how. Membrain disorder could in part explain the efficacy of cranial treatment; a gentle manual intervention to improve the housing of the right lateral frontal lobe is carried out in the hope that this will positively affect the activity or behaviour of that area of the brain.

THE AMYGDALA

On examining the anatomy of the unconscious middle brain there are two main areas where the housing of that area can be considered a factor. One is the central part of the middle brain, comprising the thalamus and limbic systems and including the amygdala. The amygdala are a pair of oval shaped structures, each about two centimetres long. They represent the brain's alarm system (reacting instantaneously to stimuli) and are involved in the laying down of unconscious memories or traces. When the amygdala are overactive, the patient will be oversensitive to triggers and this can manifest as fear, anger, aggression, anxiety, psychopathy and borderline personality disorders. When underactive, the patient will find it hard to connect or deal with people and may suffer depression and lack normal self-protective instincts.

These areas are housed in a space which is unlikely to be compressed as there are no pieces of the bony 'jigsaw puzzle' of the skull nearby, only the very dense and stable cranial base. However, it is an area that can be subject to distortion and congestion due to the proximity of the vascular (blood vessel) system and the free margins of the dura.

PITUITARY GLAND

The other part of the middle brain that needs to be considered in relation to membrain disorder is the pituitary gland. This small pea-sized gland is suspended by a stalk from the underside of the middle brain (figure 40). It fits snugly into a small bony compartment in the middle part of the cranial base. This compartment is called the pituitary fossa or cavity and is roofed over by a small membranous diaphragm, itself a continuation of the dura. The gland thus sits in a confined space that can be affected by either congestion or tension in that area and normally by a combination of the two.

Altered behaviour of the pituitary gland as a consequence of a challenging environment in the skull can manifest in both physical and emotional problems associated with hormonal imbalances. If this is the case, then the best access point to this area for a manual therapist is via the midline of the roof of the mouth. The therapist will rest a gloved finger on the palate and sense the space above it. A vertical bone called the vomer, a section of the nasal septum, connects the roof of the mouth directly to the underside of the cranial base – and from there straight up towards the pituitary fossa (figure 40).

When treating this area, it is far harder for the therapist to achieve a functional change between the vomer and the cranial base when there is an orthodontic retainer fixed behind the front teeth. This creates a vice-like compression to the whole middle face and cranial base complex. If a retainer is fitted, an osteopathic assessment would reveal whether the orthodontic work and the fixed retainer have potentially altered the behaviour of the pituitary gland. If so, then that orthodontic intervention may be responsible for some very far-reaching negative consequences.

It is important to balance this concern about the fitting of retainers with the positive consequences of a good orthodontic intervention at the right stage of life. In a child who has a very high and narrow palate the vomer has limited space. As discussed in

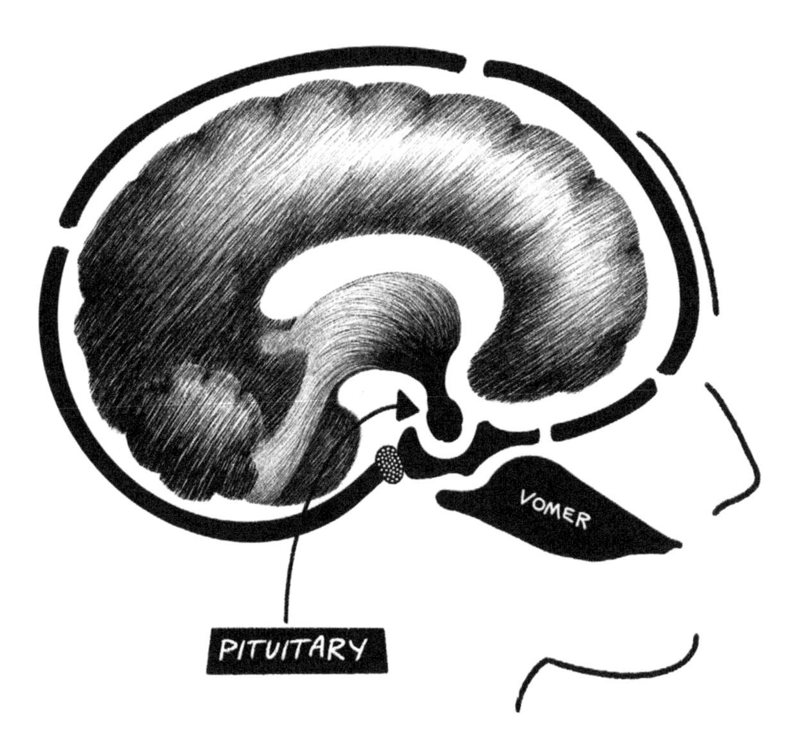

Figure 40. The pituitary and the vomer. The vomer bone sits between the roof of the mouth and the cranial base. The vomer can be examined be palpating up through the roof of the mouth.

chapter 6, there is a form of orthodontic intervention ('expansion work') which aims to expand the bony palate by putting gentle pressure laterally and forwards on the palate as it grows. The aim is to create a broad, wide and flattened palate with plenty of room for the teeth. It is a pre-emptive approach, anticipating problems of a too-crowded set of teeth. The outcome is adequate space above the palate not only for the nasal fossa but also for the vomer which in turn will promote healthy housing of the pituitary gland – all vital conditions for life-long health.

PRE-PATHOLOGICAL/PATHOLOGICAL AND THE REGIONS OF THE BRAIN

When thinking about specific areas of the brain that may be adversely affected by membrain disorder and influence mental health, it is vital to understand more about the distinction between a 'pre-pathological' and 'pathological' condition. This distinction was introduced in chapter 10: "The key to understanding health and disease is to understand in what dimension a biological system is under stress and then to understand whether the consequence of that stress is simply an adaptive change in *behaviour* at that level (a 'pre-pathological' change) or whether there has been a *structural* and irreversible reorganisation (a 'pathological' change)."

Pre-pathological

In a pre-pathological illness the *behaviour* of a system is being influenced by a challenging environment but the *structure* or *form* of the system is maintained. The change in behaviour of the system will present as symptoms. When considering general health, many readers have probably experienced feeling physically very unwell but on medical investigation such as blood tests, MRI scans, colonoscopies and so on nothing abnormal is detected. Their symptoms are a consequence of a change in the behaviour of a system (perhaps in a patient suffering with indigestion, a stomach lining that is producing too much acid) but there are no structural changes.

A pre-pathological condition is reversible. The behaviour of a system can revert to normal once the adverse environmental conditions have been corrected. In a pre-pathological condition therapeutic attention should be paid to the environment of the system, with the intention of restoring the environment to normal. A manual therapist faced with a pre-pathological condition will direct treatment towards the irrigation, nerve supply and physical housing of that system.

Pathological

In a pathological condition there has been structural change to a system, an abnormality that can be found on medical investigation. Indigestion could turn out to be a symptom of a stomach ulcer or stomach cancer. Once the structure of a system has changed, this is irreversible. In a pathological condition medical attention needs to be paid to the system itself; the ulcer or tumour has to be treated directly. This will normally require an orthodox medical intervention, as treatment will probably involve surgery, drugs or radiation.

The primary skill in diagnosing a patient lies not in giving a label to a collection of symptoms but in recognising whether a condition is pre-pathological or pathological.

The next skill is in understanding precisely when the contribution of health professionals such as manual therapists, nutritionists, medical herbalists and psychotherapists, in other words those more adept at addressing environmental conditions, will outweigh the benefit of the orthodox medical treatments – and of course vice versa.

A PATHOLOGY IN THE BRAIN

A small cancerous tumour pressing on the amygdala has been shown to lead to a complete inability to control anger, to the point that someone normally of a mild disposition may commit mass murder.[85] The growth of a cancerous tumour is a pathological change, one that cannot be reversed by improving only the environment of the brain, namely irrigation, and the state of the dura and cranial bones. A cancerous tumour means that things have gone too far; the structure of the brain has altered. Likewise, if the pituitary gland has changed its form, or the same has happened to the cerebral hemispheres, then these systems have undergone a pathological change and the condition falls outside the scope of a manual therapist. In both cases a referral to a neurosurgeon or neurologist would be indicated.

However, these are worst-case scenarios. A neglected pre-pathological condition may lead to a pathological condition. If a manual therapist in the cranial field gets involved at the pre-pathological stage, the stage of membrain disorder, pre-emptive treatment can be effective. A successful treatment will restore membrain health and this outcome will potentially have a positive impact on mood disorders, hormonal balance and the long-term condition of the brain.

IN SUMMARY

If a therapist understands which areas of the brain are implicated in different kinds of breakdown of mental health it becomes possible to target and assess the *housing* of those areas and, if an abnormality in that housing is found, to address membrain disorder and effect a change through a manual treatment – typically Balanced Membranous Tension (BMT). Supporting the dura to self-correct bony conflicts and open up constricted irrigation channels leads to a healthier environment for the brain. The brain then returns to comfortable functioning, with a consequent benefit to psychological well-being.

EIGHTEEN

A HANDS-ON THERAPEUTIC APPROACH FOR PATIENTS WITH PSYCHOLOGICAL PROBLEMS

There will be many manual therapists reading this book who will want to press the point that, without diagnosing membrain disorder as such, they nevertheless help patients with mental health problems. This is a valid point because there are many other ways in which a manual therapist can influence such patients, but the rationale and methods nevertheless differ from the approach described up to this point.

These other approaches need to be described alongside the membrain health concept so that the differences can be appreciated. The following forms of work done by manual therapists are fully warranted, documented, based on clinical trials which validate their approaches and are reinforced by respected peer-reviewed articles.

THE POWER OF TOUCH

The first discussion is around the power of touch. Touch fulfils a basic human need. There are many who derive psychological benefit from human touch, whether from a masseur, reflexologist, osteopath, craniosacral therapist, chiropractor or physiotherapist: in fact, from anyone who pays kind attention to the patient's physical body. It is a simple phenomenon and I don't want to suggest a placebo effect because it denigrates this very powerful therapeutic tool.[86,87]

PAIN RELIEF

The second discussion is around patients who are in physical pain, most commonly chronic pain, and because of the pain they become depressed or anxious. This becomes a vicious cycle where the depression makes the perception of the pain worse and so the pain-related depression becomes worse. The pain is worrying, exhausting, disabling and isolating. It may be that the manual therapist can relieve the patient of the chronic pain and as a consequence the depression or anxiety lifts.[88] A patient suffering from membrain disorder will however be living with mental health issues rather than physical pain.

PSYCHOSOMATIC CONDITIONS

The third discussion revolves around psychosomatic conditions. There is a large collection of books available on this topic. *The Body Keeps the Score* by Bessel van der Kolk and *The Body Bears the Burden* by Robert C Scaer, for instance, both describe how the body reacts both somatically (physically in the body) and biochemically (invisibly at the biomolecular level) as a response to psychological/emotional trauma.[89,90] A single traumatic event such as being raped or tortured, or a series of traumatic events, perhaps in childhood, will create long-term physical and physiological changes in the body.

A simple example of a psychosomatic condition would be a patient who is scared, perhaps a woman with an abusive husband who is constantly wary of his moods. The stress will manifest physically in her body. She will assume a protective posture, shoulders elevated and rounded, back hunched, chest protected. Her breathing will typically be shallow and fast. The resting tension of the body muscles will be higher than normal so her whole body will feel tight. She will exist in a chronic state of 'fight or flight' and the physiological response to this heightened state, which ordinarily should be short lived, carries on permanently and takes its physical and biochemical toll on her body. In some circumstances it may go the other way, so that an individual in a very stressful situation becomes almost catatonic (playing dead) in order not to attract attention.[91]

In the case of psychosomatic conditions, the problem is at the systemic level of the whole person in respect of his or her immediate environment (D5). There is a top-down effect of the environment on the physical body and the body will react.

Such a patient may well consult a manual therapist complaining of neck, back or shoulder pain. The therapist will very often detect these conditions and be able to resolve them – to some extent, or for a short time. However, this will represent 'first aid' treatment if, for example, the abusive husband is still at large. For effective treatment, the level to be targeted should be the whole person (D5), and the treatment should be talking therapy, either for the wife because of her uncomfortable home environment, to help her adapt to and deal with it, or for the husband to understand why he is being cruel to his wife and to address that behaviour. Ideally of course it would be talking therapy for the couple together, as the systemic dimension that is struggling is, in fact, the relationship of the couple.

Another and different type of psychosomatic condition has a historical origin. A *psychologically* traumatic event causes a *physical* reaction in the body at the time, one that the body somehow incorporates. It has the potential to re-emerge forcefully years later in the form of a physical ailment. An example might be of a rape that occurred decades before. This can result in a physical reaction that may exist over years yet the body has adapted to it, so the patient is unaware of it until such a time that compensations break down, perhaps due to a new stress on the body. The patient will again consult a manual therapist about their physical pain, not about a mental health issue. At this point, a well-trained practitioner with an understanding of the impact of psychological trauma on the *physical* body may recognise this chronic physical body reaction and realise that it is linked to a historical psychological trauma. Often the memory of the psychological trauma is buried away as well.

A manual therapist can work on the physical manifestation of the past psychological trauma using either direct or indirect techniques (explained in chapter 5) to effect a change. Indirect techniques (involving 'listening' to the body) are generally preferable in this situation as the process is then patient-led, so that the interventions are more guided by the patient, albeit at an unconscious level. The practitioner needs to be fully aware of what he or she is doing and, ideally, to be working alongside a talking therapist, since a historical psychological trauma harboured as a physical reaction in the body may be released during treatment. It can be a difficult time for the patient.

MEMBRAIN DISORDER VERSUS PSYCHOSOMATIC CONDITIONS

In membrain disorder the *soma* (physical structure of the body) has an effect on the *psyche* at the dimension of the brain (D4). More often than not there is no emotional trauma to be remembered. Membrain disorder is a physical condition, typically resulting from head impacts creating a response in the brain housing. Manual treatment is specifically directed towards the dura with the aim of restoring better housing and irrigation of the brain area, thus normalising the brain's behaviour. This in turn can have a positive impact on psychological health.

In contrast, in psychosomatic conditions the psyche affects the soma; emotions and associated thoughts affect the physical body. A psychosomatic condition is a 'top down effect' where the dimension of origin is at the individual level or above (D5/6). Manual treatment will be aimed at the physical effects of the patient's emotional state.

Of course membrain disorder and a psychosomatic condition can exist together if the trauma to the head had an emotional trauma attached to it – such as being mugged or involved in a traumatic car accident. It is not always clear cut. Whatever the circumstances, a manual practitioner – and the patient, if possible – should always make their best attempt at understanding which systemic dimension is being addressed by a particular treatment.

NINETEEN

A PROPOSAL

I was at the Hay Literary Festival in 2019 and mental health nurse and author Nathan Filer, a winner of the Costa prize, was being interviewed about his excellent book *The Heartland: Finding and Losing Schizophrenia.*[92] The message threaded throughout Nathan's book was that the labels, for example 'so-called schizophrenia', attached to mental health patients are inappropriate and unhelpful and – most relevantly for our purposes – do not assist the patient in securing an appropriate treatment. In the time allowed for questions after the interview it was the same recurring question from a very receptive audience – what could be done about the poor way in which people with mental health problems are diagnosed? What needed to change? For this, the author had no answer and freely but disappointedly admitted to the fact.

The decision to write this book, and in this way, was made whilst I sat in that audience.

Here is a proposal for what needs to change; what is to be done about the poor way that patients with mental health problems are diagnosed. It has been a conscious thought in my mind for nearly three decades, an idea that has become clearer over time, and the need to air it gets more and more imperative as the crisis in mental health problems escalates in the 21st century.

I am not a research scientist, a medical doctor nor a person who sits in authority. However I am a clinician who has examined and treated heads for 30 years. This is something that very few people do, nor even contemplate why they might want to do it. It is a case of 'knowledge' versus 'information' based on a long career as a manual practitioner working with a huge variety of patients and on my own further studies involving not just books and articles but also many intensive discussions with often inspirational fellow practitioners from different countries.

There are many effective and valid treatment approaches to mental health conditions and many different types of practitioners who help in different ways – a tsunami of self-help advice coming out of every media outlet. The big problem is how to direct each patient towards a therapeutic approach which is *appropriate for that individual*: one which will *help the patient to get well.*

By understanding and considering complexity and using it to identify the causative factor(s) and the biological dimension(s) of origin of a mood disorder or other mental health issue, a metaphorical 'road map' emerges. This road map can then be used to direct each individual patient presenting with mental health problems towards practitioners with the knowledge and skill set appropriate to that patient. Manual therapists trained in the cranial field and those with knowledge of membrain disorder and the skills to address it should be included in that list of practitioners.

In this book, the simple image of the Russian doll has been used to represent the six dimensions at which mental health issues may originate. For purposes of identifying the pathway to the most effective treatment, this road map needs to show not only the dimensional origin of a mental health problem but also the diagnostic methods to be employed and the range of suitable and effective treatments available (as well as a note of unsuitable approaches). It is important to embrace the idea that a singular labelled condition and its collection of symptoms as described in DSM-5, such as depression, psychosis, anxiety, OCD, and attention deficit, can originate from any one or any number of those dimensions. Symptoms are not the guide to the origin of a problem. Listening, case history, observation and palpation are the guides.

An example of a road map is offered in the Appendix.

Understanding complexity in relation to mental health diagnosis, and acknowledging the link between membrain disorder and mental health, both require mind-set changes among talking therapists and manual practitioners, patients, the medical and dental professions and the insurance and drug industries. This is not an easy thing to make happen but the first step has been writing this book and the next step is for a wide range of people to read it and express an interest in membrain health and how it sits within a new model of diagnosis designed around complexity. This wide range of people includes practitioners, patients, sports coaches, contact sports players, parents who have children with teeth braces – the list goes on.

Who knows what the next steps will be? Emergent behaviour – the inbuilt unpredictability of events – is a factor here! Diagnosing the *dimension(s) of origin* of a mental health problem, particularly the biological dimensions, is a new idea which this book adds to the already-established system of diagnosing psychological illness. The idea may be 'spat out' and the original system may maintain its original form. Alternatively, the idea may be integrated and a new system emerge.

This could have far-reaching consequences well beyond the influence of this author.

APPENDIX

A ROAD MAP TO MENTAL HEALTH DIAGNOSIS AND TREATMENT

The road map identifies three stages in diagnosis and treatment:

THE PRESENTING PROBLEM

According to Buser's eight spectrums (figure 22–29)

DIAGNOSIS OF THE CAUSATIVE DIMENSION(S)

D1–D4 biological factors, D5 & D6 social factors (figure 31)

REFERRAL TO AN APPROPRIATE THERAPIST

for treatment specifically directed at the causative dimension (D1–D6) and/or its environment

***

THE PRESENTING PROBLEM

According to Buser's eight Spectrums

1. LISTENING – Patient interview

- Patient's or carer's account of the mental health issue
- When it arose
- Perceived cause(s)
- Symptoms
- Recent/ongoing treatments and their effectiveness
- Side-effects

DIAGNOSIS OF THE CAUSATIVE DIMENSION(S)

D1–D4 Biological Factors
D5 & D6 Social Factors

2. QUESTIONING – Patient case history

- Occupation
- Family and social circumstances
- Interests and sporting history
- Lifestyle
- Past and current medical history – including accidents, operations and other physical traumas
- Past and current dental history
- Past and current emotional health history
- Past and current stress factors that they have been subject to (both physical and mental)
- Family history of mental and physical conditions

3. OBSERVATION – Physical characteristics

- Symmetry of the jaw – malocclusion
- Symmetry of the middle and upper face and the ears – plagiocephaly
- Scars – signs of physical trauma to the head, face and throat
- Condition of the skin
- Posture
- Signs of mouth breathing (open mouth posture, thin dry lips, dark rings under their eyes, increased tone of the

accessory breathing muscles that creates an anterior head posture and round shoulders)

4. PALPATION of the head
- Membrain Disorder
- Congestion

REFERRAL TO AN APPROPRIATE THERAPIST
for treatment specifically directed at the causative dimension (D1–D6) and/or its environment.

***

THE SIX DIMENSIONS OF ORIGIN

D1 BIOMOLECULAR DIMENSION

This will most likely be picked up by **LISTENING** and **QUESTIONING**.

Most commonly there will be a family history where parents, aunts, grandparents, siblings and cousins are similarly affected, perhaps on different Buser's spectrums (figs 22-29), but the common theme is an inability for relatives to maintain themselves in the functional centre of the various spectrums. In these situations there is generally a genetic basis causing a lifelong imbalance in the neuroendocrine system. It is a structural and irreversible condition and therefore it is important to target treatment directly at the biomolecular level. This requires psychotropic drugs which are prescribed by a psychiatrist.

These patients need the kind attention of a psychiatrist.

Note: If the causative dimension of a patient's psychological problem is above D1, there will be a 'top-down' effect which will alter the balance of the neuroendocrine system (D1). Symptoms may ease with the prescribing of psychotropic drugs. However the ***cause*** *(anywhere above D1) is not being directly addressed by drugs aimed at D1. Such treatment in these circumstances can only be described as 'First Aid'.*

D2 CELLULAR DIMENSION

This will most likely be picked up in the **QUESTIONING, OBSERVATION** and **PALPATION** stages. The focus will be on assessing the health of the connective tissue system that supports the cellular dimension.

QUESTIONING will show up whether a patient has a poor diet, lives or works in a toxic environment, or if they drink, smoke or take too many recreational drugs. These patients are not getting the correct nutrients and are putting toxins into their system. Questioning will also tell whether the patient is getting enough exercise, fresh air and sunshine.

OBSERVATION will show whether the patient is getting insufficient oxygen into their system due to poor breathing. It will show in the condition of the skin. Acne, cysts, pallor and dryness are an indication of the health of the general connective tissue system. It is the same connective tissue matrix that supports the neurones.

PALPATION can give clues as to whether there is an efficient irrigation system operating within the confines of the cranium. A poor irrigation system will compromise the delivery of oxygen and nutrients and the removal of waste products. There will be congestion that builds over time. If there is generalised congestion within this confined space, it is palpable. The head will feel full and heavy and the quality of the membrain system poor and unexpressive. It is a very distinctive feel.

All of the above problems are reversible. If a depleted and toxic neuronal environment can be restored to a healthy and less challenging environment this will affect the behaviour of the neurones in a positive way.

The appropriate **treatment** for an issue originating at D2 would be a combination of:

- dietary and lifestyle advice (nutritionist, medical herbalist, dietician, life coach and other reputable practitioners who can help improve the cellular environment).
- teaching of good breathing techniques (yoga teacher and breathing specialist), exercise (personal trainer).
- fresh air and sunshine (self-help).
- support for the liver and kidneys (nutritional, supplements or detox).
- a manual intervention aimed at improving the micro-circulation of fluid through the closed cavity of the cranium (manual therapist trained in the cranial field).

Some patients suffering with their mental health are unable to breath properly because of a deviated nasal septum, swollen adenoids and tonsils. All of these situations are structural and can be irreversible and may require a surgical intervention (ear nose and throat specialist). Other patients with poor breathing habits may have a very high narrow palate which compromises the passage of air through the nose and into the lungs. Again this is a structural condition and requires a direct orthodontic intervention (functional orthodontist).

The mass of self-help advice available on every possible media platform and the array of nutritionists, breathing experts, personal trainers and hands-on therapists suddenly becomes more navigable. There are many different elements contributing to a common problem. By identifying the specific element(s) involved it is easier to target the best therapeutic or self-help approach.

Note: If the causative dimension of a patient's psychological problem is D5 or D6 (individual/social) then addressing the health of the connective tissue matrix (D2) will not address the ***origin*** *of their problem. There is no doubt that everyone will benefit from a healthy connective tissue matrix in terms of their general health. There will always be top-down and bottom-up effects from achieving a healthy connective tissue matrix. However if a patient's issues arise from going through a traumatic divorce (D5), or the patient is suffering because of lockdown restrictions during a global epidemic (D6) or the patient has a genetic condition affecting the balance of his or her neuroendocrine system (D1) all the measures described above will not directly address the* ***origin*** *of their problem.*

D3 MULTICELLULAR DIMENSION

This will most likely be picked up in the **LISTENING** and **QUESTIONING** stages.

LISTENING

Patients suffering at the dimension D3 will typically have symptoms commonly associated with the label of PTSD.

QUESTIONING

They will present with some sort of traumatic history which has meant neuronal circuits associated with that trauma keep firing even though the danger has passed. These patients relive the emotional effects of the trauma over and over again, triggered by the slightest of stimuli.

The appropriate treatment in these circumstances is to try to desensitise the relevant circuit.

Psychotherapists have a collection of tools that they are trained to use. The obvious ones for a D3 issue would be EMDR, CBT, or music or art therapy. Hypnotists may be able to help.

If the patient is locked into a cycle of high alertness this will affect the tadpole-shaped membrain system (the dura) which becomes fixed into a long narrow shape. It is possible with a hands-on approach for a manual therapist to release the 'tadpole' out of this shape. This will give the nervous system a chance to self-reset. However this will be a short-term fix unless other measures specifically suited to D3 are used alongside this approach.

Self-help practices such as meditation, Tai chi or Qigong could work at this dimensional level.

D4 THE BRAIN

This will most likely be picked up from **QUESTIONING, OBSERVATION** and **PALPATION**.

QUESTIONING will reveal whether a patient had a traumatic birth or has subsequently suffered a head or pelvic trauma as a child, teenager or adult. It will reveal whether they played contact sports and for how long and to what level. It will reveal if they have had orthodontic or major dental interventions or whether they have had face or jaw surgery.

OBSERVATION will show if they have a distortion in the face or jaw caused by a malocclusion or plagiocephaly or both. Frown lines and asymmetrical wrinkles, in the older patients, can offer clues to underlying long-term problems in the skull.

PALPATION is the ultimate decider as to whether a patient is suffering with membrain disorder. A patient may have an asymmetrical face, had years of orthodontic treatment, played rugby for twenty years and fallen out of a tree when he was a child, but if the membrain system is not distorted, it has no story to tell. Then it will be clear to the practitioner that the body has resolved old traumas, compensated effectively around any legacies remaining and membrain disorder is *not* a factor in the patient's mental health problem.

Conversely, if all the questioning or observation does not suggest a membrain disorder, but on palpating the skull a distortion in the underlying membrain system is detected, then it is possible that membrain disorder *is* a contributing factor to the patient's mental health problem. The environment of the brain is affecting the brain's behaviour and compromising the irrigation system of the brain, threatening its long-term health. In this case the patient needs a hands-on approach from a suitably trained osteopath, chiropractor or physiotherapist.

If there are pathological (irreversible) changes to the brain such as CTE, the accumulation of tau proteins in the brain tissue, dementia, etc., it is possible that a hands-on approach may slow down the deterioration but fundamentally these patients will now need to be under the care of a neurologist or neuropathologist.

Note: If the causative dimension of a patient's psychological problem is D1, D2, D3, D5 or D6 and they receive a hands-on treatment to the cranium, the patient will be relaxed by the treatment and probably derive some short-term benefit from it. However the origin of their condition is not being addressed.

D5/D6 THE WHOLE PERSON

This will most likely be picked up by **LISTENING** and **QUESTIONING**. It may be that the patient is experiencing, or has previously lived through, difficult times – painful circumstances and events in their life. In these cases the whole person has either to find a way to change their environment or to adapt to that which cannot be changed. These patients need a talking therapist.

There will always be top-down and bottom-up effects. A difficult time going through a relationship break-up will have a top-down effect resulting in different parts of the brain (D4) becoming over- or under-active and an imbalance in the neuroendocrine system (D1). The same difficult experience will have a bottom-up effect on other relationships the patient has with children, friends or workmates (D6). But it is the dimension of the whole person (D5) in relationship with their environment, past and present, that needs to be addressed if the causative dimension is to be targeted directly, and for this a talking therapist is appropriate.

An exception would be where there has been a past emotional trauma and the impact of that emotional trauma on the physical body has not been resolved. In that case it might be that a manual therapist would be useful to consult as well, but only alongside the talking therapist.

SUMMARY

When mental health patients are prescribed psychotropic drugs for their DMS-5 labelled symptoms, they are being treated directly at the biomolecular dimension (D1). The biomolecular level is being significantly altered by elements (drugs) added to the system. This will create a 'bottom-up effect' and emergent behaviour will be the consequence, rippling up the dimensions in unpredictable ways. The possible extent of this is evident in the long list of 'side-effects' accompanying every drug.

When a patient consults a talking therapist they are usually being treated at the level of the individual (D5) in relation to their environment (relationships, work situation, etc.). The talking therapist is dealing here with the 'top down' effects. Other treatment approaches employed by talking therapists are directed at the multicellular dimension (D3), for example CBT, EMDR, and art or music therapy.

When considering the dimensions visualised as the Russian

doll it is clear that the biomolecular (D1), the multicellular (D3) the individual (D5) and society (D6) dimensions are considered by the doctors and psychotherapists but not necessarily differentiated in regard to which treatment a patient should receive.

There is a lot of attention being paid to the brain (D4) by the neuroscientists (as opposed to the practitioners) via the exciting advances being made in neuroimaging – seeing the brain in action. Thomas Insel, a prominent neuroscientist, professes that all mental problems have a biological origin in the brain.[93] It is impossible to deny this. However, when the Dimensional Model is taken into account it could be argued that the brain, while always involved, is not necessarily the dimension of *origin* of the mental anguish. Part One of this book offered a new understanding of the impact of the many different types of head trauma on mood disorders and brain degenerative diseases.

To recognise that membrain disorder can be a causative factor in mental health problems allows for specifying when the brain (D4) might in fact be the dimension of origin of the patient's suffering. This understanding might lead into a new avenue of discussion and research which will help sports people and others subjected to head trauma – worldwide.

Many patients suffering psychological anguish originating at the biological levels D1–D4 are from happy families, they may live comfortably with no serious financial worries, they may have no other significant health problems – but their mental suffering is as real as anyone else's.

The intention of both Part One and Part Two of this book is to help these people and their therapists to identify at which biological level they might be suffering. Then they can be directed towards an effective treatment or a suitably orchestrated combination of treatments.

GLOSSARY

Alzheimer's disease – a form of dementia (meaning a decline of brain functioning). It can affect memory, thinking skills and other mental abilities.

Amino acids – biomolecules that are the building blocks of proteins.

Anatomy – the identification and description of the structures of living things. It is a branch of biology and medicine.

Arachnoid mater – the middle layer of the three-layer membrane system that surrounds the brain and spinal cord.

Art therapy – the British Association of Art Therapists defines art therapy as "a form of psychotherapy that uses art media as its primary mode of expression and communication".

Attachment points of the skull – areas where the dura condenses and binds to the inside of the skull at particular places.

Autism – a complex, lifelong developmental disability that typically appears during early childhood and can impact a person's social skills, communication, relationships, and self-regulation. Autism is defined by a certain set of behaviours and is a 'spectrum condition' that affects people differently and to varying degrees.

Balanced Membranous Tension (BMT) technique – a manual therapy approach by a practitioner trained in the cranial field aiming to interact with the dural membrane and bring it to a point of 'no tension'. It is at this point of no tension that the membrane system can reorganise itself.

Biomolecules – the most essential organic or complex molecules, involved in the maintenance and metabolic processes of living organisms.

Bipolar disorder – previously known as manic depression, is a condition that affects moods, which can swing from one extreme to another.

Brain hemisphere – the forebrain or cerebral brain is divided by a groove into two parts, the left and right hemisphere (meaning half-sphere).

Broca's area – an area of the lateral frontal lobe in the dominant hemisphere, usually the left, concerned with the production of speech.

CBT – See Cognitive Behavioural Therapy.

Cell – the basic structural, functional, and biological unit of all known organisms. A cell is the smallest unit of life.

Central nervous system (CNS) – the part of the nervous system consisting of the brain and spinal cord.

Cerebral cortex – the forebrain. It is made of white and grey matter and is divided anatomically into lobes known as the frontal, parietal, occipital and temporal lobes.

Cerebral palsy – a problem that affects muscle tone, movement, and motor skills. It hinders the body's ability to move in a coordinated and purposeful way. It is a non-inherited neurological condition caused by brain damage to the cerebral cortex.

Cervical spine – the seven vertebrae of the neck.

Chiropractor – a manual therapist who treats problems primarily of the bones, muscles and joints.

Chronic Traumatic Encephalopathy (CTE) – a degenerative brain condition associated with repeated blows to the head, typically found in boxers and players of contact sports.

Coccyx or 'tailbone' – the triangular bony structure located at the very bottom of the spine (the evolutionary remnant of a tail).

Cognitive Behavioural Therapy (CBT) – a type of psychotherapeutic treatment that helps people learn how to identify and change destructive or disturbing thought patterns that have a negative influence on behaviour and emotions.

Compensatory mechanism – any means by which the body adapts itself to a region of the body that is not fully functioning.

Complex system – a non-living system of increasingly complex systemic levels.

Complex adaptive system – a living system composed of increasingly complex systemic levels, for example a human being. Each level will adapt its behaviour in order to maintain itself in changing environmental conditions. A level unable to maintain itself will either disintegrate into its component parts (i.e. degenerate and die) or it will replicate.

Complexity theory – a contemporary scientific approach which seeks to understand complicated systems such as climate, economics, digital systems or societies through interactions and the feedback loops these generate.

Compulsions – see Obsessive Compulsive Disorder.

Concussion – temporary unconsciousness or confusion caused by an impact to the head.

Consciousness – an ill-defined term. It is used to refer to (i) the waking state, awareness, (ii) experience; and (iii) the possession of any mental state.

Contact sports – a sport in which the participants necessarily come into bodily contact with one another. Some are scored on impacting another e.g. boxing and mixed martial arts, some on body tackling e.g. rugby, American football, Australian football, and some via incidental or deliberate contact with sports equipment e.g. hockey or lacrosse, heading in soccer.

Contributory factor – one of a number of underlying reasons for a patient to experience symptoms. Several contributory factors can act in combination to cause a person to be unwell.

Cranial base (also known as base of skull, skull base; latin: *basis cranii*) – part of the skull forming the floor of the cranial cavity. The base bones are the ethmoid, sphenoid and part of the occiput and temporal bones.

Cranial cavity – the space inside the cranium that houses the brain and associated soft tissue and vascular structures.

Cranial osteopath (also known as an osteopath trained in the cranial field) – an osteopath (see below) who uses an 'indirect' approach towards the whole body and the head.

Cranial vault – The superior (higher) part of the skull forming the roof and sides of the cranial cavity. The vault bones are the frontal, parietals and upper parts of the occiput, temporals and sphenoid.

Cranium (also known as the skull) – the hard bone case that gives an animal's or a human's head its shape and protects the brain.

CTE – see Chronic Traumatic Encephalopathy.

Cysts – sac-like pockets of membranous tissue containing fluid, air, or other substances.

Degenerative brain disease – a progressive degeneration or death of neurons (brain cells) and brain matter over time affecting many of the body's activities, such as balance, movement, talking, breathing, heart function, memory and personality. It includes many named medical conditions such as Dementia, Parkinson's and CTE.

Dementia – an umbrella term for a range of conditions that affect the brain, with symptoms such as memory loss, speech difficulties and confusion that become worse over time. There are more than 200 sub-types such as Alzheimer's, vascular dementia and frontotemporal dementia. Dementia can occur at any age but is more common in people over 65.

Digestive system – the tube passing from the mouth to the anus and associated organs such as the lungs and pancreas.

Dura, or Dura mater – (also known as the dural membrane) is a double layered membrane which forms the outermost membranous covering of the brain and spinal cord within the skull. It also divides the cranial cavity into compartments. It is part of the continuous fascial system of the body.

Ectoderm – the upper layer of the embryonic disc that will develop into the central nervous system and skin.

Embryo – early stage of development of a multicellular organism. In humans it refers to the stage between 2 and 9 weeks, the portion of the life cycle that begins just after fertilization and continues through the formation of tissues and organs.

Embryonic disc – a pear-shaped structure composed of three distinct layers: the ectoderm, mesoderm and endoderm; the initial form of the embryo. It is at this stage in development that the orientation of the developing human form is determined – a left and right side, a front and back and a top and bottom.

EMDR – see Eye Movement Desensitisation & Reprocessing.

Emergent behaviour – appears when a number of simple entities (agents) operating in an environment come together to form more complex *behaviours*. The *emergent* property itself may be either very predictable, or unpredictable and unprecedented, and can represent a new level of the system's evolution.

Endoderm – the lower layer of the embryonic disc that will develop into the future digestive system and associated organs.

Entropy – the second law of thermodynamics which describes how isolated systems spontaneously evolve towards thermodynamic equilibrium, the state with maximum entropy.

Eye Movement Desensitisation & Reprocessing (EMDR) – a form of cognitive behavioural therapy in which the therapist guides the patient to think about a past trauma while moving the eyes back and forth, left to right. Over time, this helps the brain to reprocess the memories so that they cause less pain.

Fascia (also referred to as membrane) – a form of connective tissue that forms sheet-like coverings around organs, vessels and the musculoskeletal system.

Feedback loop – part of a biological system in which some portion (or all) of the system's output is used as information for future response and maintenance of the same system. There can be positive and negative feedback loops.

Fluid irrigation system – all areas of the body are irrigated at the micro, meso and macro level. Fluids at the macro level move via blood and lymph channels but there is also movement of fluids outside of these vessels, between the cells and in and out of the cells.

Frontal lobe – the frontal lobe of the brain lies behind the forehead (frontal bone) and processes what it is to be human in the form of consciousness, awareness. It enables the recognition of 'I', identity, self-will and decision-making.

Functional orthodontists – orthodontists who use mouth appliances to expand the bones of the middle and lower face to make more room to accommodate the teeth, to improve the way the teeth fit together (the occlusion) and to open up the airway system.

Gene – the basic physical and functional unit of heredity. In biology, a gene is a sequence of nucleotides in DNA or RNA that encodes the synthesis of a gene product, either RNA or protein.

Genetic inheritance – genes that are passed down through the generations. If the genes are faulty this fault may pass down from parents to children.

Hormones – chemical messengers secreted directly into the blood, which carries them to organs and tissues of the body to exert their effects.

Immune system – the responsive system that protects your body from harmful substances, germs and cell changes that could make you ill. It is made up of various organs, cells and proteins and serves a vital function.

Impulse control problems – a condition in which a person has trouble controlling emotions or behaviours. Often, the behaviours violate the rights of others or conflict with societal norms and/or the law.

Indirect approach – a manual approach used in osteopathy which works gently with the 'pulls' of the soft tissue structures (muscles, fascia, dura) to encourage reflex changes such that tension in the structures is released.

Limbic system – a set of structures located in the midbrain that deals with emotions and memory. It regulates autonomic or endocrine function in response to emotional stimuli and is also involved in reinforcing behaviour.

Lipids – biomolecules that are the building blocks of fats and of phospholipids (essential for the formation of cell membranes).

Malocclusion – an irregular bite, or meeting of the teeth.

Manual therapist – someone who treats people using a hands-on approach, such as an osteopath, chiropractor, masseur, or reflexologist.

Mesoderm – the middle layer (inner tissue) of the embryonic disc. It receives information and nutrition from the mother's womb and delivers it to the upper and lower layers of the embryonic disk.

MRI scan – a type of scan that uses strong magnetic fields and radio waves to produce detailed images of the inside of the body, including the soft tissues, organs, the brain, muscles, and vertebral discs.

Musculoskeletal problems – symptoms and conditions arising from the bones, muscles and ligaments anywhere in the body.

Music therapy – an established psychological clinical intervention delivered by registered music therapists. It helps people whose lives have been affected by injury, illness or disability, through supporting their psychological, emotional, cognitive, physical, communicative, and social needs.

Neuroendocrine system – a complex regulatory mechanism that includes the hypothalamus, the pituitary and its connections to the midbrain, and their combined control over the body's entire endocrine system.

Neuroimaging (brain imaging) – the use of various techniques to image, directly or indirectly, the structure and function of the nervous system. It is a relatively new discipline within medicine, neuroscience, and psychology.

Neurotransmitters – chemical messengers that transmit a message from a nerve cell across the synapse to a target cell. The target can be another nerve cell, a muscle cell or a gland cell. Neurotransmitters are chemicals generated by the nerve cell specifically to transmit the message.

Non-pathological – a change in *behaviour* of a system ('illness') but not a change of its *form* or *structure*. Non-pathological conditions are reversible with the right treatment. See Pathological.

Nucleotides – biomolecules that are the building blocks of DNA (deoxyribonucleic acid).

Obsessive Compulsive Disorder (OCD) – has two main elements: obsessions and compulsions. *Obsessions* are unwelcome thoughts, images, urges, worries or doubts that repeatedly appear in the mind, generating anxiety or mental discomfort. *Compulsions* are repetitive activities carried out to reduce the anxiety caused by the obsession, such as repeatedly checking that a door is locked or constantly repeating a phrase in one's head.

Occlusion – how the upper and lower teeth meet – the bite. See Malocclusion.

Orthodontist – a dental specialist who deals with misalignment of the teeth and the jaw using dental braces and other appliances to alter the position of the teeth and jaws.

Orthodox medicine – the conventional art and science of the diagnosis and treatment of disease and the maintenance of health, conforming with generally accepted standards of practice. It is practised by medical doctors and their support staff – radiographers, nurses, physiotherapists, and many others.

Orthognathic surgery – corrective jaw surgery addresses conditions of the jaw and face related to structure, growth, sleep apnoea, TMJ disorders, malocclusion problems or other orthodontic problems that cannot easily be treated with braces. Also used to treat congenital conditions such as cleft palate. Typically during oral surgery, bone is cut, moved, modified, and realigned.

Osteopath – a manual practitioner who uses an osteopathic philosophy of diagnosis and treatment for a wide range of medical conditions. An osteopath works with the physical structures of the body to restore motion where absent. According to the osteopathic philosophy, without motion, nutrients and oxygen cannot be supplied to an area and waste products cannot be removed. This creates a predisposition to disease. To restore motion is to provide the optimum conditions for the body to self-correct, to self-heal, and to maintain health.

Outside-inside phenomenon – the behaviour of a system is dependent on environmental conditions (the system's housing). When environmental conditions change, the system will change its behaviour in the effort to maintain itself.

Palate – roof of the mouth.

Palpation – a method of feeling with the fingers or hands as part of a physical examination. Skilled palpation can determine the size, form, consistency, texture, location, and tenderness of an organ or body part.

Paranoia – thinking and feeling of being threatened in some way, when there is little or no evidence. Paranoid thoughts can also be described as delusions. There are different kinds of threat a person might be scared and worried about.

Parietal lobe – the parietal lobes are situated at the top of the brain and are mainly concerned with movement. The right parietal lobe holds a 'whole' living body image – an affective (emotional) experience of oneself. A person with damage in this area may be disconnected and cut off.

Parkinson's disease – a condition which affects the brain. It causes symptoms such as shaking and stiffness that worsen over time.

Pathological change – a clinical finding by a pathologist where there is an infection, a change found in tissue cultures or on organ examination.

Phrenology – literally study of the mind; the study of the shape of the *skull* as indicative of *mental* faculties and character traits. It became a popular pursuit in the nineteenth century, reflecting European attempts to link morality, character and intelligence to race, gender, class and genetics. While phrenology is discredited, modern studies confirm that different mental functions are located in specific areas of the brain.

Physical legacies – unresolved strain patterns from old injuries; the body adapts around them. They may be mild and unproblematic but can become significant when the body has to adapt to new injuries.

Physiological system – the human body comprises trillions of physiological systems, from intracellular systems operating on a molecular level to the highly developed central nervous system (CNS). In complexity and size, these systems range from those contained within the cell to those responsible for coordinating the activity of millions of cells. Yet, each shares the common purpose of regulating different aspects of the body's functions so that homeostasis (balance) is maintained.

Physiotherapy – physiotherapists work within the orthodox medical system and help people affected by injury, illness or disability, through movement and exercise, manual therapy, education and advice. They are often involved in rehabilitation following accidents or medical treatment.

Pia mater – the inner layer of the three-layer membrane system (dura) that covers the brain and spinal cord.

Plagiocephaly – medical term for an uneven or asymmetrical head shape.

Post-concussion syndrome – a complex disorder in which various symptoms such as headaches, dizziness and pain last for weeks and sometimes months after the injury that caused the concussion.

Post-natal – the period after birth.

Predisposing factor – an underlying cause which explains why one patient my develop a health issue and another person under similar conditions may not. For example, an old injury to a hip may result in early arthritic changes in that hip many years later.

Psychiatrist – a physician or medical doctor who specialises in psychiatry, the branch of medicine devoted to the study, diagnosis, treatment and prevention of mental disorders.

Psychologist – a specialist in normal and abnormal mental states, perceptual, cognitive, emotional, and social processes and behaviour. Psychologists may assess an individual's psychological health within family, school, workplace and other social settings, or as research psychologists experiment with, observe, record and interpret how individuals relate to one another and to their environments.

Psychosis – a symptom of a disorder in the way the brain processes information. It causes a loss of touch with reality, resulting in seeing, hearing, or believing things that are not real to others around them.

Psychotherapist – a person who treats mental disorders by psychological rather than medical means.

Psychotropic drug – any drug that affects behaviour, mood, thoughts, or perception. Medically approved psychotropic drugs are prescribed to treat a variety of mental health issues which significantly impair healthy functioning.

Retainers (dental) – appliances designed to hold teeth in place once an orthodontic procedure to alter their position is complete. They may be 'temporary' (a mouthguard slotted over the teeth and often worn at night), or 'permanent' (a hidden wire fixed behind the teeth).

Saccharides – biomolecules that are the building blocks of sugars.

Schizophrenia – the name given to a psychiatric disorder characterized by continuous or relapsing episodes of psychosis. Major symptoms include hallucinations (often hearing voices), delusions, and disorganized thinking. Other symptoms include social withdrawal, decreased emotional expression, and apathy.

Sciatica – a nerve pain that can affect the whole or part of a lower limb, including the foot. It is caused by constant or intermittent pressure at some point on the main nerve passing from the spine through the hip muscles down to the leg.

Scoliosis – sideways curvature of the spine.

Sick building syndrome – a common worldwide health concern, describing how people in a building suffer from symptoms of illness or become infected with chronic disease induced by the building in which they work or reside.

Sociopath – the defining characteristic of the sociopath is a profound lack of *conscience* – an absence, due to a brain disorder, of the 'moral compass' that steers most people away from breaking common rules and towards treating others decently. Sociopaths frequently have a charming demeanour, are cunning, have an excessive sense of self-worth and are pathological liars.

Sutures – the joint lines between the individual bones of the skull. There are many different designs of suture in a single skull.

System – any self-organised form able to maintain itself within its environment.

Systems theory – the interdisciplinary study of systems, whether natural or man-made. It seeks to understand how systems, comprising a range of interacting elements, behave in time and space (see also Complexity Theory).

Tau proteins – proteins that help to stabilise the internal skeleton of neurons (nerve cells) in the brain.

Temporal bones – a pair of bones that form the side walls of the cranial vault and the lateral aspects of the cranial base. They house the hearing and balancing apparatus and nerves inside the bone, the bony channels through which blood passes into and out of the cranial fossa, and the lateral poles of attachment for the dura. Each temporal bone has complex sutural connections with seven neighbouring bones that constitute the metaphorical '3-D jigsaw puzzle' of the skull.

Temporal lobe – a part of the cerebral hemisphere located under the temporal bone.

Tensegrity – a principle found in nature and used in architecture and design in which compression elements are balanced by a tensile (stretching) force. In the body, bones are held in position by tension from muscles and fascia rather than by any rigid structure.

Trauma – a medical term for any significant injury or group of injuries, physical and/or emotional, which have a serious adverse impact on an individual. In ordinary speech (UK) 'trauma' normally means an emotionally distressing experience.

Traumatic Brain Injury (TBI) – damage caused to the brain from an external mechanical force. TBI is classified according to severity (from 'mild traumatic brain injury' to 'severe traumatic brain injury'), on mechanism ('non-penetrating' or 'penetrating' head injury), or other features such as occurring in a specific location or over a widespread area. TBI can result in physical, cognitive, social, emotional and behavioural symptoms while outcomes can range from complete recovery to permanent disability or death.

Venous (blood) sinus system – it is located within the two layers of the dura and manages the drainage of blood from the confines of the skull into blood vessels which transport it through the neck and back to the heart.

Viscero-cranium – the facial skeleton.

Vomer – a vertical bone, a section of the nasal septum (the cartilage and bone in the nose), which connects the roof of the mouth directly to the underside of the cranial base.

X-ray – types of electromagnetic radiation best known for their ability to see through a person's skin and reveal images especially of the bones beneath it.

ENDNOTES

1 Few osteopaths today seem aware of Still's lifelong interest in mental health. In 1917 a letter about the Still-Hildreth Sanatorium in Macon, Missouri, was found by his deathbed. Still spoke of "progress that is being made … in the treatment of mental and nervous disease.… My personal experience covers a period of something over fifty years in the treatment of mental cases.… I have always contended that a majority of the insane patients could be successfully treated by osteopathy … and I am very anxious for the entire profession to know of the work that is being done." Lewis, J. R. (2012) *A. T. Still: From the Dry Bone to the Living Man*. Blaenau Ffestiniog, Wales: Dry Bone Press, p. 354

2 Sutherland, G. S. *Teachings in the Science of Osteopathy* edited by Anne L. Wales. Portland, OR: Rudra Press 2003 (1990)

3 The cranium is viewed in the Monro-Kellie doctrine as a closed box containing three compartments, the 1400g brain (85%), 50–75ml of blood (about 5%), and 150ml of cerebrospinal fluid (10%), which are incompressible. On inter-cranial pressure see Tameem, A. & Krovvidi, H. (2013). Cerebral physiology. *Continuing Education in Anaesthesia Critical Care & Pain* Vol. 13, Issue 4, pp. 113–118. https://doi-org.ucc.idm.oclc.org/10.1093/bjaceaccp/mkt001

4 Engel, G. L. (1977). The Need for a New Medical Model: A Challenge for Biomedicine. *Science*, New Series, Vol. 196, No. 4286, pp. 129–136 DOI: 10.1126/science.847460 https://www.jstor.org/stable/1743658 (accessed 1 Apr 2022)

5 For an asessment of Engel's influence forty years on, see Fava G, A. & Sonino N., (2017). From the Lesson of George Engel to Current Knowledge: The Biopsychosocial Model 40 Years Later. *Psychotherapy*

and Psychosomatics. Vol. 86, pp. 257–259. DOI: 10.1159/000478808

6 Bordoni, B., Simonelli, M. & Lagana, M. M. (2019). Tentorium Cerebelli: Muscles, Ligaments, and Dura Mater, Part 1. *Cureus*. 11(9): e5601. https://doi.org/10.7759/cureus.5601

7 Aylwin, M. (2021). Head injury is the silent killer, players don't know whether they have it. *The Guardian*, 18 April. https://www.theguardian.com/sport/2021/apr/18/kyran-bracken-head-injury-is-the-silent-killer-concussion-sport-rugby-union (accessed 8 Nov 2021)

8 Siva, N. (2020). Scotland to ban heading in children's football. *The Lancet*, Vol. 395, Issue 10220, p. 258, January 25. https://doi.org/10.1016/S0140-6736(20)30118-5

9 Gouttebarge, V., Hopley, P., Kerkhoffs, G., Verhagen, E., Viljoen, W., Wylleman, P. & Lambert, M. I. (2017). Symptoms of Common Mental Disorders in Professional Rugby: An International Observational Descriptive Study. *International Journal of Sports Medicine*. 38(11), 864–870. DOI: 10.1055/s-0043-114010

10 Lee, B., Bennett, L. L., Bernick, C., Shan, G. & Banks, S. J. (2019). The Relations among Depression, Cognition, and Brain Volume in Professional Boxers: A Preliminary Examination Using Brief Clinical Measures. *Journal of Head Trauma Rehabilitation*. November/December 2019, Vol. 34, Issue 6, pp. E29–E39. https://doi.org/10.1097/HTR.0000000000000495

11 Goldschmidt, H. (2018). Brain Injuries in Sport: Remedies Under English Law. 17 October. https://www.morgansl.com/en/latest/brain-injuries-sport-remedies-under-english-law (accessed 13 Feb 2022)

12 Dale, M. and Smith, M. R. (2021). Retired Black Players Fight NFL Brain Injury Payout Algorithm Based on Race. *Insurance Journal*. 18 May. https://www.insurancejournal.com/news/national/2021/05/18/614610.htm (accessed 13 Feb 2022)

13 Maroon, J. C., Winkelman, R., Bost, J., Amos, A., Mathyssek, C. & Miele, V. (2015). Chronic Traumatic Encephalopathy in Contact Sports: A Systematic Review of All Reported Pathological Cases. *PLoS ONE* 10(2): e0117338. https://doi.org/10.1371/journal.pone.0117338 and "correction" at https://journals.plos.org/plosone/article?id=10.1371/journal.pone.0130507 (accessed 5 Mar 2022)

14 Joshi, S. M. (2008). The sick building syndrome. *Indian Journal of Occupational and Environmental Medicine*. Vol. 12, Issue 2, pp. 61–64. https://doi.org/10.4103/0019-5278.43262

15 Redlich, C. A., Sparer, J. & Cullen, M. R. (1997). Sick-building syndrome. *The Lancet*, Vol. 349, Issue 9057, pp. 1013–1016, April 05.

https://doi.org/10.1016/S0140-6736(96)07220-0

16 Baltazir, G.A., Kolwitz, K., Petrone P., Stright, A. & D'Andrea, J. (2020) Osteopathic Manipulative Treatment Relieves Post-concussion Symptoms in a Case of Polytrauma. *Cureus* 12(3): e7317. doi.org/10.7759/cureus.7317

17 Guernsey, D.T., Leder, A. & Yao, S. (2016). Resolution of Concussion Symptoms after Osteopathic Manipulative Treatment: a Case Report. *Journal of the American Osteopathic Association.* Mar; 116(3): e13–7. DOI: 10.7556/jaoa.2016.036

18 Castillo, I., Wolf, K. & Rakowsky, A (2016). Concussions and Osteopathic Manipulative Treatment: An Adolescent Case Presentation. *Journal of the American Osteopathic Association.* Mar; 116(3): 178–181. DOI: 10.7556/jaoa.2016.034

19 The experience of former England scrum-half Kyran Bracken is recounted in Aylwin, M.(2021) Kyran Bracken: Head injury is the silent killer, players don't know whether they have it. *The Guardian,* 18 April. https://www.theguardian.com/sport/2021/apr/18/kyran-bracken-head-injury-is-the-silent-killer-concussion-sport-rugby-union (accessed 8 Nov 2021)

20 Willer, B. S., Zivadinov, R., Haider, M. N., Miecznikowski, J. C. & Leddy, J. J. (2018). A Preliminary Study of Early-Onset Dementia of Former Professional Football and Hockey Players. *Journal of Head Trauma Rehabilitation.* September/October, Vol. 33, Issue 5, pp. E1–E8. DOI: 10.1097/HTR.0000000000000421

21 Lee, B., Bennett, L. L., Bernick, C., Shan, G. & Banks, S. J. (2019). The Relations Among Depression, Cognition, and Brain Volume in Professional Boxers: A Preliminary Examination Using Brief Clinical Measures. *Journal of Head Trauma Rehabilitation.* Vol. 34, Issue 6, pp. E29–E39. https://doi.org/10.1097/HTR.0000000000000495

22 Penke, L., Bates, T. C., Gow, A. J., Pattie, A., Starr, J. M., Jones, B. C., Perrett, D. I. & Deary, I. J. (2009). Symmetric faces are a sign of successful cognitive aging. *Evolution and Human Behavior.* Vol. 30, 6, November, pp. 429–437. https://doi.org/10.1016/j.evolhumbehav.2009.06.001

23 Schleip, R., Jäger, H. & Klingler, W. (2012). 4.2 – Fascia is alive: How cells modulate the tonicity and architecture of fascial tissues. In Schleip, R., et al. *Fascia: The Tensional Network of the Human Body.* London: Churchill Livingstone, pp. 157–164. https://doi.org/10.1016/B978-0-7020-3425-1.00057-X

24 Schleip, R., Jäger, H., & Klingler, W. (2012). What is 'fascia'? A review of different nomenclatures. *Journal of Bodywork and Move-*

ment Therapies. Vol. 16 (4), pp. 496–502. https://doi.org/10.1016/j.jbmt.2012.08.001

25 Mackinlay, A., Grace, R., Horwood, J., Fergusson, D. & MacFarlane, M. (2009). Adolescent psychiatric symptoms following preschool childhood mild traumatic brain injury: evidence from a birth cohort. *Journal of Head Trauma Rehabilitation*. May–Jun; 24(3): pp. 221–7. DOI: 10.1097/HTR.0b013e3181a40590

26 Richard, Y. F., Swaine, B. R., Sylvestre, M. P., Lesage, A., Zhang, X. & Feldman, D. E. (2015). The Association between Traumatic Brain Injury and Suicide: Are Kids at Risk? *American Journal of Epidemiology*. Volume 182, Issue 2, 15 July, Pages 177–184. https://doi.org/10.1093/aje/kwv014

27 McHugo, G. J., Krassenbaum, S., Donley, S., Corrigan, J. D., Bogner, J. & Drake, R. E. (2017). The Prevalence of Traumatic Brain Injury among People with Co-Occurring Mental Health and Substance Use Disorders. *Journal of Head Trauma Rehabilitation*. 32(3), May/June, pp. E65–E74. https://doi.org/10.1097/HTR.0000000000000249

28 Wasserman, L., Shaw, T., Vu, M., Ko, C., Bollegala, D. & Bhalerao, S. (2008). An overview of traumatic brain injury and suicide. *Brain Injury*. Vol. 22, Issue 11, pp. 811–819. https://doi.org/10.1080/02699050802372166

29 Mackelprang, J. L., Harpin, S. B., Grubenhoff, J. A.,& Rivara, F. P. (2014). Adverse Outcomes Among Homeless Adolescents and Young Adults Who Report a History of Traumatic Brain Injury. *American Journal of Public Health*. Vol. 104, Issue 10, pp. 1986–1992. https://doi.org/10.2105/AJPH.2014.302087

30 McMillan, T. M. Graham, L., Pell J. P., McConnachie, A. & Mackay, D. F. (2019). The lifetime prevalence of hospitalised head injury in Scottish prisons: A population study. *PLoS ONE* 14(1): e0210427. https://doi.org/10.1371/journal.pone.0210427

31 Korinthenberg, R., Schreck, J., Weser, J., & Lehmkuhl, G. (2004). Post-traumatic syndrome after minor head injury cannot be predicted by neurological investigations. *Brain & Development*. Vol. 26, Issue 2, Mar., pp. 113–117. https://doi.org/10.1016/S0387-7604(03)00110-4

32 Griauzde, J. & Srinivasan, A. (2018). Advanced Neuroimaging Techniques; Basic Principles and Clinical Applications. *Journal of Neuro-Ophthalmology*. Volume 38, Issue 1, pp. 101–114. https://doi.org/10.1097/wno.0000000000000539

33 Wager, T., Barrett, L. F., Bliss-Moreau, E., Lindquist, K., Duncan, S., Kober, H., Joseph, J., Davidson, M. and Mize, J. (2008). The Neu-

roimaging of Emotion. Ch. 15 in: Lewis, M., Haviland-Jones, J. and Barrett, L. F. *Handbook of Emotions*. 3rd edition. London: The Guilford Press, pp. 249–271. Available at: https://www.researchgate.net/profile/Tor-Wager/publication/284430179_The_neuroimaging_of_emotion/links/5ad4de45458515c60f546102/The-neuroimaging-of-emotion.pdf (accessed 1 Apr 2022)

34 The cranium is viewed in the Monro-Kellie doctrine as a closed box containing three compartments, the 1400g brain (85%), 50–75ml of blood (about 5%), and 150ml of cerebrospinal fluid (10%), which are incompressible. On inter-cranial pressure see Tameem, A. & Krovvidi, H. (2013). Cerebral physiology. *Continuing Education in Anaesthesia Critical Care & Pain*. Vol. 13, Issue 4, pp. 113–118. https://doi-org.ucc.idm.oclc.org/10.1093/bjaceaccp/mkt001

35 Carter, R. (2010). *Mapping the Mind*. London: Weidenfeld and Nicolson. Ch. 8 "Higher Ground" pp. 295–336.

36 Weinberger, D. R., Aloia, M. S., Goldberg, T. E. & Berman, K. F. (1994). The frontal lobes and schizophrenia. In *Journal of Neuropsychiatry and Clinical Neurosciences*. Vol. 6, Issue 4, pp. 419–427. (Published correction in Vol. 7, Issue 1, p. 121). https://doi.org/10.1176/jnp.6.4.419

37 Williams, M. R., Chaudhry, R., Perera, S., Pearce, R. K. B., Hirsch, S. R., Ansorge, O., Thom, M. & Maier, M. (2013). Changes in cortical thickness in the frontal lobes in schizophrenia are a result of thinning of pyramidal cell layers. *European Archives of Psychiatry and Clinical Neuroscience*. 263, pp. 25–39. https://doi.org/10.1007/s00406-012-0325-8

38 Çiçek, M., Gitelman, D., Hurley, R. S. E., Nobre, A. & Mesulam, M. (2007). Anatomical Physiology of Spatial Extinction. *Cerebral Cortex*. Vol. 17, Issue 12, December, pp. 2892–2898. https://doi.org/10.1093/cercor/bhm014

39 Davidson, R. J., Putnam, K. M. & Larson, C. L. (2000). Dysfunction in the Neural Circuitry of Emotion Regulation – A Possible Prelude to Violence. *Science*. Vol. 289, No. 5479, pp. 591–594. DOI:10.1126/science.289.5479.591

40 Tobia, K. P. (2017). Phineas Gage. *Reference Module in Neuroscience and Biobehavioral Psychology*. Elsevier: Science Direct. https://doi.org/10.1016/B978-0-12-809324-5.03144-8

41 Collins, M. (2016). *The British School of Osteopathy: The First 100 Years*. Bloomington, IN: Xlibris UK. The front cover shows the shield and motto of the School from the 1950s.

42 See e.g. Nestor, J. (2020). *Breath: The New Science of a Lost Art*. Lon-

don: Penguin Life

43 Kiyak, H. A., McNeill, R. W. & West, R. A. (1985). The emotional impact of orthognathic surgery and conventional orthodontics. *American Journal of Orthodontics and Dentofacial Orthopedics*. Vol. 148, Issue 6, pp. 1054–1066. https://doi.org/10.1016/S0002-9416(85)90217-9

44 Kojima, T., Yoshizawa, M., Ono, Y., Kurabe, K., Kano, H., Saito, C. & Kobayashi, T. (2015). Three Cases of a Mental Disorder Appearing after Orthognathic Surgery. *Journal of the Japanese Socety of Jaw Deformities*. Vol. 25, Issue 3, pp. 230–240. https://doi.org/10.5927/jjjd.25.234

45 Fleming, P. S. & Flood, T. R. (2005). Steroid-induced psychosis complicating orthognathic surgery: A case report. *British Dental Journal*. Vol. 199, pp. 647–648. https://doi.org/10.1038/sj.bdj.4812929

46 Businesswire (Jan 12, 2022). Global Orthodontic Consumables Market Research Report (2021 to 2027) – by Product, Patient, Equipment, End-user and Region – ResearchAndMarkets.com https://www.businesswire.com/news/home/20220112005547/en/Global-Orthodontic-Consumables-Market-Research-Report-2021-to-2027---by-Product-Patient-Equipment-End-user-and-Region---ResearchAndMarkets.com (accessed 8 Feb 2022)

47 Scarr, G. (2008). A model of the cranial vault as a tensegrity structure, and its significance to normal and abnormal cranial development. *International Journal of Osteopathic Medicine*. Vol. 11, Issue 3, pp. 80–89. https://doi.org/10.1016/j.ijosm.2008.03.006

48 Strolling under the Skin – Dr. Jean-Claude Guimberteau (video). https://www.youtube.com/watch?v=ky0BmGP5nbU (accessed 4 May 2022)

49 Cannon, M., Jones, P. B. & Murray, R. M. (2002). Obstetric Complications and Schizophrenia: Historical and Meta-Analytic Review. *The American Journal of Psychiatry*. Vol. 159, pp. 1080–1092. https://doi.org/10.1176/appi.ajp.159.7.1080

50 World Health Organization (no date). Child Maltreatment. https://www.who.int/news-room/fact-sheets/detail/child-maltreatment (accessed 10 Mar 2022)

51 Olson, B., Ustanko, L. & Warner, S. (1991). The Patient in a Halo Brace: Striving for Normalcy in Body Image and Self-Concept. *Orthopaedic Nursing*. Vol. 10, Issue 1, pp. 44–50. https://doi.org/10.1097/00006416-199101000-00009

52 NHS (2018). Causes – Post-traumatic stress disorder. https://www.nhs.uk/conditions/post-traumatic-stress-disorder-ptsd/causes/

(accessed 9 Nov 2021)
53 E.g. National Institute of Mental Health, USA (2020). Why do some people develop PTSD and other people do not? Post-Traumatic Stress Disorder (online). https://www.nimh.nih.gov/health/publications/post-traumatic-stress-disorder-ptsd (accessed 9 Nov 2021)
54 Kamm, O. (2021). *Mending the Mind: The Art and Science of Overcoming Clinical Depression*. London: Weidenfeld & Nicolson, p.14
55 Bodkin, H. (2017). Doctors 'too reliant' on depression questionnaire designed by Pfizer, campaigners warn. *The Telegraph*, 21 May. https://www.telegraph.co.uk/news/2017/05/21/doctors-reliant-depression-questionnaire-designed-bypfizer-campaigners/ (accessed 9 Nov 2021)
56 Pincus, T., de C Williams, A. C., Vogel, S. & Field, A. (2004). The development and testing of the depression, anxiety, and positive outlook scale (DAPOS). *Pain*. 109, Issue 1, pp. 181–188. https://doi.org/10.1016/J.PAIN.2004.02.004
57 McGilchrist I. (2011). The Divided Brain – Iain McGilchrist. Ted-ed video. https://www.ted.com/talks/iain_mcgilchrist_the_divided_brain
58 American Psychiatric Association (2021). DSM History. https://www.psychiatry.org/psychiatrists/practice/dsm/history-of-the-dsm
59 Davies, J. (2013). *Cracked: Why Psychiatry is Doing More Harm Than Good*. London: Icon Books
60 Filer, N. (2019). *The Heartland: Finding and Losing Schizophrenia*. London: Faber & Faber
61 Buser, S. with Cruz, L. (2014). *DSM-5 Insanely Simplified: Unlocking the Spectrums within DSM-5 and ICD-10*. Asheville, NC: Inner Quest, p.27
62 Chui, G. (2000). Unified Theory Is Getting Closer, Hawking Predicts. *The Mercury News* (San Jose), January 23, p. 29A
63 Basios, V. (2017) The Century of Complexity: Dr Vasileios Basios talks to Jane Clark and Michael Cohen about new ideas in science. *Beshara Magazine*. Issue 6, Summer. https://besharamagazine.org/science-technology/dr-vasileios-basios-the-century-of-complexity/ (accessed 9 Nov 2021)
64 Engel, G. L. (1977). The Need for a New Medical Model: A Challenge for Biomedicine. *Science. New Series*, Vol. 196, No. 4286, pp. 129–136. DOI: 10.1126/science.847460 https://www.jstor.org/stable/1743658 (accessed 9 Mar 2022)
65 Fava G, A. & Sonino N., (2017). From the Lesson of George Engel to Current Knowledge: The Biopsychosocial Model 40 Years Lat-

er. *Psychotherapy and Psychosomatics*. Vol. 86, pp. 257–259. DOI: 10.1159/000478808

66 Benning, T. B. (2015). Limitations of the biopsychosocial model in psychiatry. *Advances in Medical Education and Practice*. Vol. 6, pp. 347–352. https://www.ncbi.nlm.nih.gov/pmc/articles/PMC4427076 (accessed 9 Mar 2022)

67 Phillips, J. (2017). What is Entropy – Jeff Phillips. Ted-ed video. https://www.youtube.com/watch?v=YM-uykVfq_E (accessed 9 Nov 2021)

68 Fields, R. D. (2011). The Hidden Brain. *Scientific American Mind*. May. https://doi.org/10.1038/scientificamericanmind0511-52

69 Pollack, G. H. (2013). The Fourth Phase of Water: A role in fascia? *Journal of Bodywork and Movement Therapies*. Vol. 17, Issue 4, October, pp. 510–511. https://doi.org/10.1016/j.jbmt.2013.05.001

70 Insel, T. R. (2010). Faulty Circuits. *Scientific American*. Vol. 302, Issue. 4, pp. 44–51. https://doi.org/10.1038/scientificamerican0410-44

71 McLaughlin, K. A., Weissman, D. & Bitrán, D. (2019). Childhood Adversity and Neural Development: A Systematic Review. *Annual Review of Developmental Psychology*. Vol. 1, pp. 277–312. https://doi.org/10.1146/annurev-devpsych-121318-084950

72 Amen, D. (2011). Daniel Amen – Change Your Brain, Change Your Life. TedXOrange Coast video. Available at https://www.youtube.com/watch?v=MLKj1puoWCg (accessed 12 Feb 2022)

73 Decker, M. & Fleischer, T. (2008). Contacting the brain – aspects of a technology assessment of neural implants. *Biotechnology Journal*. Vol. 3, Issue 12, Special issue: Brain Matters, pp. 1502–1510. https://doi.org/10.1002/biot.200800225 (accessed 9 Nov 2021)

74 For the test and results calculator see e.g. the MDCalc PHQ-9 (Patient Health Questionnaire 9) page at https://www.mdcalc.com/phq-9-patient-health-questionnaire-9 (accessed 1 Apr 2022)

75 See e.g. Andalo, D. (2016) Antidepressants associated with increased risk of suicidal thoughts in healthy adults. *The Pharmaceutical Journal*, 17 October. https://www.pharmaceutical-journal.com/news-and-analysis/news/antidepressants-associated-with-increased-risk-of-suicidal-thoughts-in-healthy-adults/20201834 article reporting on Bielefeldt A. Ø, Danborg P. B. & Gøtzsche, P. C. (2016) Precursors to suicidality and violence on antidepressants: systematic review of trials in adult healthy volunteers. *Journal of the Royal Society of Medicine*. Vol. 109, Issue 10, pp. 381–392. doi: 10.1177/0141076816666805

76 Council for Evidence-Based Psychiatry, Ed. (2019) New Study: an-

tidepressants significantly raise the risk of suicide in the treatment of depression for adults, 25 June. http://cepuk.org/2019/06/25/new-study-antidepressants-significantly-raise-risk-suicide-treatment-depression-adults/ reporting on Hengartner, M. P. & Plodel, M. (2019). Newer-Generation Antidepressants and Suicide Risk in Randomized Controlled Trials: A Re-Analysis of the FDA Database. *Psychotherapy and Psychosomatics*. Letter to the Editor, Vol. 88, pp. 247–248. https://doi.org/10.1159/000501215

77 Boseley, S. (2000) Happy drug Prozac can bring on impulse to suicide, study says. *The Guardian*, 22 May. https://www.theguardian.com/science/2000/may/22/drugs.uknews reporting the work of David Healy. See Healy, D. (2000). Emergence of antidepressant induced suicidality. *Primary Care Psychiatry*. Issue 6, pp. 23–28. https://davidhealy.org/wp-content/uploads/2012/05/2000-Healy-Healthy-Volunteer-Suicide.pdf (accessed 9 Nov 2021)

78 Tchernegovski, P., Reupert, A. & Maybery, D. (2014). "Let's Talk about Children": A pilot evaluation of an e-learning resource for mental health clinicians. *Clinical Psychologist*. Vol. 19, Issue 1, pp. 49–58. DOI https://doi.org/10.1111/cp.12050

79 Carter, R (2010) *Mapping the Mind*. London: Weidenfeld and Nicolson, Chapter 1 "The Emerging Landscape" pp. 34–35

80 Peter, S. (2012). *The Chimp Paradox: The Mind Management Programme for Confidence, Success and Happiness*. London: Vermilion – Penguin Books

81 Insel, T. R. (2010). Faulty Circuits. *Scientific American*. Vol. 302, Issue. 4, pp. 44–51. https://doi.org/10.1038/scientificamerican0410-44

82 Bechara, A., Damasio, A. R., Damasio, H. & Anderson, S. W. (1994). Insensitivity to future consequences following damage to human prefrontal cortex. *Cognition*. Vol. 50, Issues 1–3, April–June 1994, pp. 7–15. https://doi.org/10.1016/0010-0277(94)90018-3

83 Majdandžić, J., Amashaufer, S., Hummer, A., Windischberger, C. & Lamm, C. (2016). The selfless mind: How prefrontal involvement in mentalizing with similar and dissimilar others shapes empathy and prosocial behavior. *Cognition*. Vol. 157, December, pp. 24–38. https://doi.org/10.1016/j.cognition.2016.08.003

84 Decety, J., & Michalska, K. J. (2010). Neurodevelopmental changes in the circuits underlying empathy and sympathy from childhood to adulthood. *Developmental Science*. Vol. 13, Issue 6, November, pp. 886–899. https://doi.org/10.1111/j.1467-7687.2009.00940.x

85 Carter, R (2010) *Mapping the Mind*. London: Weidenfeld and Nicolson, Chapter 4 "A Changeable Climate" pp. 149–150

86 Smith, D. W., Arnstein, P., Rosa, K. C. & Wells-Federman, C. (2002). Effects of Integrating Therapeutic Touch into a Cognitive Behavioral Pain Treatment Program: Report of a Pilot Clinical Trial. *Journal of Holistic Nursing*. Vol. 20, Issue 4, pp. 367–87. https://doi.org/10.1177/089801002237593
87 Monroe, C. M. (2009). The Effects of Therapeutic Touch on Pain. *Journal of Holistic Nursing*. Vol. 27, Issue 2, pp. 85–92.https://doi.org/10.1177/0898010108327213
88 Linton, S. J. & Bergbom, S. (2011). Understanding the link between depression and pain. *Scandinavian Journal of Pain*. Vol. 2, Issue 2, pp. 47–54. https://doi.org/10.1016/j.sjpain.2011.01.005
89 Van der Kolk, B. (2014). *The Body Keeps the Score: Brain, Mind, and Body in the Healing of Trauma*. London: Viking
90 Scaer, R. C. (2014). *The Body Bears the Burden: Trauma, Dissociation, and Disease*. London: Routledge
91 Porges, S. W. (2001). The polyvagal theory: phylogenetic substrates of a social nervous system. *International Journal of Psychophysiology*. Vol. 42, Issue 2, October, pp. 123–146. https://doi.org/10.1016/S0167-8760(01)00162-3
92 Filer, N. (2019). *The Heartland: Finding and Losing Schizophrenia*. London: Faber & Faber
93 Insel, T. R. (2010). Faulty Circuits. *Scientific American*. Vol. 302, Issue. 4, pp. 44–51. https://doi.org/10.1038/scientificamerican0410-44

ACKNOWLEDGMENTS

This book has been developing in my head over the last three decades. It was the Covid-19 lockdown in March 2020 that finally gave me the head space and the time to transfer my thoughts and ideas onto paper. It has been a steep learning curve but a gratifying one. It is something I could not have done without the cumulative input that I have received from so many people over those decades – patients, teachers, friends, and friends of friends. The amount of support that I have been offered during the process of writing has been beyond anything imaginable.

I would like to thank (in chronological order!):

Nick Woodhead for first showing me the awe-inspiring beauty of the bones of the skull which ignited in me a life-long passion.

Carol Plumridge, for not only her skilled hands in treating me, but in showing me the extraordinary impact a treatment of the skull can have on mental health.

The late Robin Kirk, principal of the London School of Osteopathy, who taught me "osteopathy in its intended format" years after I graduated as an osteopath. It was only after long discussions with Robin alongside my studies in the cranial field that I grasped that osteopathy is not about treating the musculoskeletal system, it was about using the musculoskeletal system as a tool to treat the whole body – to have a far-reaching impact on the health of the whole body. Work became so much more interesting at that point. Robin wholeheartedly supported me in my writing although he has sadly missed the book. I have missed his counsel through this process. I have missed him.

Fiona Walsh who offered me so many wonderful opportunities at an early stage of my career by recommending me as a lecturer to teach "osteopathy in the cranial field" at a number of colleges abroad. Consequently, I had the chance to travel and work, broadening my horizons in so many ways. It culminated in my becoming a member of the faculty of the Vienna School of Osteopathy (WSO) for twelve years. The school employed teaching faculty from all over the world and I got to spend time with them, talking to them, learning from them – many are still friends to this day.

I would also like to thank the students I taught at the WSO; they inspired me – their intelligence, acceptance and inquiry into intuitive medicine, some of them medical doctors who had become dissatisfied with the prescriptive nature of their own work. They questioned me, challenged me, they gave so much time and dedication to their studies, most of them working full time and raising families alongside their studies. We were all inspired by one another and by osteopathy. It was hard work but it was a joyful time.

Jean Paul Hoeppner ('JP'), Max Girardin and the Evolutionary Osteopathy fellowship (EvOst) – a big resounding thank you! It was in travelling to Belgium and meeting and studying under Max and JP that I finally found my 'osteopathic home'. I had left WSO after twelve years of teaching osteopathy in the cranial field as I was unsatisfied with the explanations and language that I myself was using and I wanted to advance my own studies. Max and JP's teaching provided many answers and the framework to hang all my thoughts and ideas on. Part two of the book is based on their teaching – their work, their explanation, their foundations for explaining health and disease in a different way – they are both brilliant heretics with decades of intense study and clinical experience behind them. I hope above all hopes that they approve of the way that I have explained 'systems and environments, chronology and complexity' although I am convinced they will find fault. They are famously discerning and extremely difficult to please!

My patients – I would like to thank the many patients who have put their trust in me. I hope I have deserved it. This book is an explanation of my rationale of treatment. I hope such treatment will become more understood, accepted and available to everyone who might need it. To any observer watching an osteopath trained in the cranial field it looks like 'faith healing' or 'magic' but it is not. It is a *skill* learnt and mastered over years and decades. It is not a cure-all or an answer to everyone's problems but it is a potent therapeutic intervention that is currently undervalued and misunderstood.

My patient editor Prof. Brian Bocking – words fail me in expressing my gratitude. Brian has given me so much time, advice, counsel, support, ideas, criticism (in the kindest way) and encouragement. He has believed in me and in the book. There have been times when I have metaphorically speaking thrown the book in the bin (difficult when everything is electronic now and held in shared files) but he has metaphorically speaking picked the book back out again and looked after it until he has nudged me back into action. Thank you, Brian.

I would like to thank my eleven anonymous book reviewers who took the time to read and give frank and honest feedback on the whole book when it was still at a very early stage. I wonder if you still recognise it? Your feedback was invaluable and acted upon.

I would also like to thank David Boyle, Sue Holliday, Paul Stead and Liz Page for their support, brainstorming, ideas and encouragement offered at crucial stages.

Hugo Russell, thank you for your wonderful illustrations. It has been a pleasure to sit alongside you and watch you re-create my terrible attempts at drawings into something quite beautiful.

Finally, I would like to thank my friend Mimi Harris. Mimi offered me 'refuge in a storm' so that, in troubled times, I was able to focus on my writing. I have felt her support every step of the way.

ILLUSTRATIONS

I am grateful to Dr Ann McKee, Boston University School of Medicine for permission to reproduce the image of the scan of the skull of Aaron Hernandez (figure 6) and to Chiron Press for permission to reproduce the text and drawings illustrating the eight spectrums of psychological health in Steven Buser's *DSM-5 Insanely Simplified* (figs 22-29).

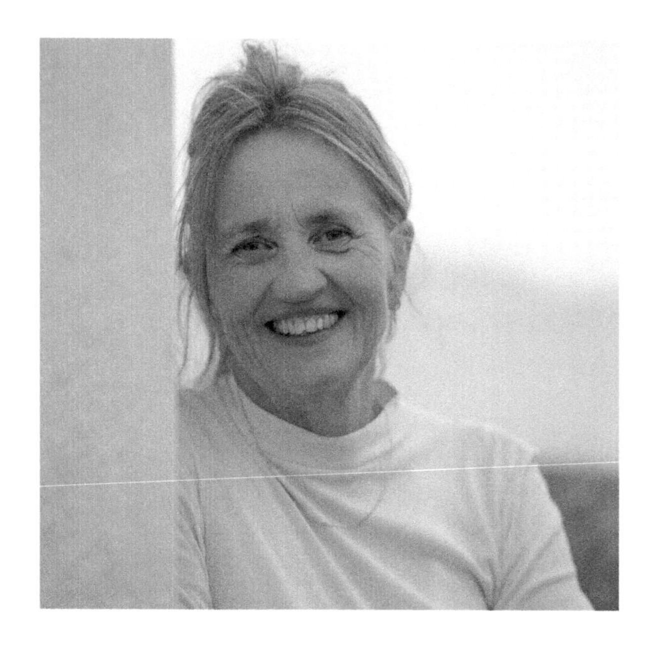

JO WILDY is a highly regarded cranial osteopath who has practised, taught and examined widely in the UK and abroad. Originally a geneticist, she has for the past 30 years successfully used osteopathic methods to treat thousands of patients, including many with mental health issues including unexplained anxiety and depression.

www.jowildy.com